Developing
Clinical
Competence

A Workbook for the **OTA**

Developing Clinical Competence

A Workbook for the **OTA**

Marie J. Morreale, OTR/L, CHT
Adjunct Faculty
Rockland Community College
State University of New York
Suffern, New York

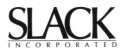

www.Healio.com/books

ISBN: 978-1-61711-815-9

Developing Clinical Competence: A Workbook for the OTA includes ancillary materials specifically available for faculty use. Please visit www.efacultylounge.com to obtain access.

Marie J. Morreale has no financial or proprietary interest in the materials presented herein.

The procedures and practices described in this publication should be implemented in a manner consistent with the professional standards set for the circumstances that apply in each specific situation. Every effort has been made to confirm the accuracy of the information presented and to correctly relate generally accepted practices. The authors, editors, and publisher cannot accept responsibility for errors or exclusions or for the outcome of the material presented herein. There is no expressed or implied warranty of this book or information imparted by it. Care has been taken to ensure that drug selection and dosages are in accordance with currently accepted/recommended practice. Off-label uses of drugs may be discussed. Due to continuing research, changes in government policy and regulations, and various effects of drug reactions and interactions, it is recommended that the reader carefully review all materials and literature provided for each drug, especially those that are new or not frequently used. Some drugs or devices in this publication have clearance for use in a restricted research setting by the Food and Drug and Administration or FDA. Each professional should determine the FDA status of any drug or device prior to use in their practice.

Any review or mention of specific companies or products is not intended as an endorsement by the author or publisher.

SLACK Incorporated uses a review process to evaluate submitted material. Prior to publication, educators or clinicians provide important feedback on the content that we publish. We welcome feedback on this work.

Published by: SLACK Incorporated
                 6900 Grove Road
                 Thorofare, NJ 08086 USA
                 Telephone: 856-848-1000
                 Fax: 856-848-6091
                 www.Healio.com/books

Contact SLACK Incorporated for more information about other books in this field or about the availability of our books from distributors outside the United States.

Printed in the United States of America.

Last digit is print number: 10 9 8 7 6 5 4

Dedication

This book is dedicated to OTA students everywhere, with the hope it will help you to succeed as you enter the wonderful world of occupational therapy.

Contents

Developing Clinical Competence: A Workbook for the OTA includes ancillary materials specifically available for faculty use. Please visit www.efacultylounge.com to obtain access.

Acknowledgments

A number of people deserve thanks for their assistance with this project. I will always be grateful to Ellen Spergel, past coordinator of the Occupational Therapy Assistant (OTA) Program at Rockland Community College, for giving me a start in academia. Her wisdom, kindness, and support regarding OTA education have impacted me forever. I would especially like to thank Donna Knoebel, coordinator of the OTA Program, for her support of this project and expertise in the area of mental health. Her input was invaluable for Chapter 6. Appreciation goes to Kathy Babcock and Mae Eng for their knowledge regarding different practice areas. I am also grateful to Debbie Amini and Randy Marti for being my "go-to" people whenever I had a clinical question during this endeavor. I admire their amazing breadth of knowledge and professional accomplishments, and appreciate their many helpful suggestions. Debbie's commitment to the profession and her leadership regarding the promotion of "occupation" will influence practitioners and students for many years to come. I am honored she took the time to review a number of exercises in this book, and I appreciate her insight, inspiration, and friendship. My OTA students deserve thanks for providing feedback when completing many of the worksheets. A special mention goes to Brien Cummings at SLACK Incorporated for his help in bringing my vision for this book to fruition.

In addition, my son, Michael, deserves recognition for helping me upgrade my technology skills. Finally, special thanks to my husband, Richard, for enduring many take-out meals and allowing me to monopolize the computer. Without his love, patience, and support, this book would not have been possible.

Marie J. Morreale, OTR/L, CHT

About the Author

Marie J. Morreale, OTR/L, CHT has more than 15 years of experience teaching occupational therapy assistant (OTA) students at Rockland Community College, State University of New York in Suffern. As an adjunct faculty member in the OTA program, Marie currently teaches Professional Issues and Documentation and Geriatric Principles. Over the years she also taught several other courses in the OTA program, including Occupational Therapy Skills, Advanced Occupational Therapy Skills, Therapeutic Activities, and Advanced Therapeutic Activities. Marie has made significant contributions to curriculum development and also served as interim coordinator of the OTA Program.

Marie graduated Summa Cum Laude from Quinnipiac College (now Quinnipiac University) in Hamden, Connecticut. She has experience working in a variety of occupational therapy practice settings including inpatient and outpatient rehabilitation, long-term care, adult day care, home health, cognitive rehabilitation, and hand therapy. Marie has been a Certified Hand Therapist for 20 years and also served several years on a home health professional advisory committee, consulting on quality assurance issues. Marie has co-authored two OTA textbooks: *The OTA's Guide to Documentation: Writing SOAP Notes, Third Edition* and *The OTA's Guide to Writing SOAP Notes, Second Edition*. In addition, she has written a chapter on documentation for *The Occupational Therapy Manager, Fifth Edition*; published several occupational therapy articles; and is the author of two online continuing education courses. Marie is active in her church community and enjoys anything travel related.

Introduction

How to Use This Book

This workbook is designed to help occupational therapy assistant (OTA) students and novice practitioners develop the "practical" problem-solving and "real-life" skills essential for fieldwork and clinical practice. The workbook is intended as a user-friendly resource to help the reader apply occupational therapy concepts and improve the clinical reasoning skills needed for academic coursework and successful transition to fieldwork and entry-level practice. The worksheets, learning activities, and suggested worksheet answers are written in an easy-to-read format and include a variety of methods such as multiple choice, matching, and true/false questions; case studies; vignettes; fill in the blanks; and experiential activities. Competencies are broken down into smaller units and explained step-by-step to allow for easy independent study. This manual will help the reader work through a wide range of situations commonly encountered in occupational therapy for various practice areas. Many helpful tips are presented to guide the OTA in proper clinical decision making, professional conduct, and meeting standards of care. Although the chapters and exercises are presented in a logical progression, each chapter is fully independent of the others. Thus, the reader can skip around and complete individual chapters or particular exercises in the order most conducive to one's individual learning needs. The book can be used as a companion text for multiple classes throughout an OTA curriculum. Many of the exercises can be used to help measure attainment of knowledge for specific educational standards delineated by the Accreditation Council for Occupational Therapy Education (ACOTE, 2012). The worksheets and learning activities are also useful as role playing exercises, studying in small groups, or as a useful study aid when preparing for fieldwork or the national certification exam. Thoroughly explained worksheet answers are provided so that readers can check their responses with suggested best practice.

The instructional methods, learning activities, and worksheets presented in this book stem from the author's more than 15 years of experience teaching OTA students. Included are topics such as professionalism; ethical behavior; effective communication; roles and responsibilities; supervision; interventions for a variety of conditions, situations, and practice areas; assessment of client function; safety; documentation; group process; evidence-based practice; and more. Many of the questions and learning activities were developed to specifically address common mistakes or difficulties exhibited by OTA students during their academic coursework and fieldwork—so that you can avoid making the same errors. As you complete the exercises in this manual, the information presented will help you to understand and apply important concepts and techniques, problem solve situations step by step, organize and prioritize interventions, improve clinical reasoning, demonstrate professional behaviors, and communicate more effectively. "Answers" to the worksheet exercises are explained clearly and simply at the end of each chapter. However, as it is impossible to present or predict every possible scenario or intervention, realize that these answers are often suggestions of best practice. It is possible that other best practice examples you come up with may also be correct. This workbook is not meant to be a book on theory, nor an instruction manual for technical hands-on skills. Thus, it is expected that the reader will have some basic knowledge of occupational therapy theory. Readers should utilize pertinent resources as needed to fill in any personal gaps in knowledge or physical skills that may become apparent when completing exercises in this workbook.

Guiding Principles

The specific roles and responsibilities of the occupational therapist (OT) and OTA in the areas of evaluation, intervention, and outcomes are delineated in the American Occupational Therapy Association's (AOTA) *Guidelines for Supervision, Roles, and Responsibilities During the Delivery of Occupational Therapy Services* (2009) and *Standards of Practice for Occupational Therapy* (2010c). The OTA works under the supervision of an OT and partners with the OT to perform selected, delegated tasks for which the OTA demonstrates service competency and is in accordance with state and federal regulations (AOTA, 2009, 2010a). Considering that each client is unique with individual circumstances, OTs and OTAs use a holistic, client-centered approach. A variety of methods and interventions are implemented to work toward the goal of contributing to a client's or population's occupational performance as described in the *Occupational Therapy Practice Framework: Domain and Process* (AOTA, 2014) and *Scope of Practice* (AOTA, 2010b). The services that occupational therapy practitioners provide are also guided by the *Occupational Therapy Code of Ethics and Ethics Standards* (AOTA, 2010a), relevant laws, facility policies, third-party payer requirements, and evidence-based practice.

While this book presents sound guidelines, an occupational therapy practitioner must always use clinical judgment to determine the methods, interventions, or recommendations that are most appropriate for a client's personal situation. OTs and OTAs must carefully consider the client's medical status and circumstances; specific client factors, contexts, and skills that hinder or support performance; any precautions or contraindications; safety issues; available methods; and current evidence supporting clinical practice. It is important to realize that a "standard" intervention for a particular condition, such as a specific physical agent modality, splint, exercise protocol, communication strategy, or adaptive device, may not be appropriate for all clients with the same diagnosis. Also, an intervention plan might delineate more than one device or method as a particular kind of intervention (i.e., a condition that requires splinting may necessitate using both a nighttime static positioning splint and a daytime dynamic mobilization splint).

The scenarios presented are representative of situations commonly encountered in clinical practice. The names and specific details have been fabricated to create optimal learning exercises, so any specific resemblance to an actual person is purely coincidental. It is the author's intent that this book will be a useful resource to help the OTA student succeed in school and become a competent practitioner. Any feedback or suggestions for future editions is welcome.

References

Accreditation Council for Occupational Therapy Education. (2012). 2011 Accreditation Council for Occupational Therapy Education (ACOTE) standards. *American Journal of Occupational Therapy, 66*(6 Suppl.), S6-S74. doi: 10.5014/ajot.2012.66S6

American Occupational Therapy Association. (2009). Guidelines for supervision, roles, and responsibilities during the delivery of occupational therapy services. *American Journal of Occupational Therapy, 63*(6), 797-803. doi: 5014/ajot.63.6.797

American Occupational Therapy Association. (2010a). Occupational therapy code of ethics and ethics standards (2010). *American Journal of Occupational Therapy, 64*(6 Suppl.), S17-S26. doi: 10.5014/ajot.2010.64S17

American Occupational Therapy Association. (2010b). Scope of practice. *American Journal of Occupational Therapy, 64*(6 Suppl.), S70-S77. doi: 10.5014/ajot.2010.64S70

American Occupational Therapy Association. (2010c). Standards of practice for occupational therapy. *American Journal of Occupational Therapy, 64*(6 Suppl.), S106-S111. doi: 10.5014/ajot.2010.64S106

American Occupational Therapy Association. (2014). Occupational therapy practice framework: Domain and process (3rd ed.). *American Journal of Occupational Therapy, 68*(1 Suppl.), S1-S48. doi: 10.5014/ajot.2014.682006

Chapter

1

Communicating Effectively

Good verbal and nonverbal communication skills are essential traits for occupational therapy practitioners. This chapter presents worksheets and learning activities to help you problem solve, practice, and respond appropriately to common situations with clients, families, significant others, caregivers, and other professionals. Practical communication tips are provided to help you make a good first impression, explain your role effectively to different audiences, ask open-ended questions, actively listen, and show empathy. Suggested answers to worksheet exercises are provided at the end of the chapter.

Contents

Morreale, M. J.
Developing Clinical Competence: A Workbook for the OTA (pp. 1-27).
© 2015 SLACK Incorporated.

Worksheet 1-1

Initial Client Encounter

Mary, an occupational therapy assistant (OTA), is meeting her client, Jane Doe, for the first time. Jane is 80 years old and sustained a right cerebrovascular accident 1 week ago, resulting in left hemiparesis. Jane was recently admitted to a skilled nursing facility for rehabilitation and requires moderate assistance for self-care and transfers. Consider Mary and Jane's initial conversation below. What suggestions would you make regarding the OTA's interaction with the client?

OTA: Hey Jane, I'm Mary, your therapist for today. It is nice to meet you. Any problems?
Client: Yes, my TV isn't working and my breakfast was late this morning. Who are you again?
OTA: I'm your OTA for today and I am here to help you get dressed.
Client: What's an OTA?
OTA: Well, I'm from the occupational therapy department. We are similar to physical therapy, except they work on walking and the lower extremities and we work on the upper extremities and activities of daily living—ADLs. Are you ready to begin therapy now sweetie?

Suggestions to improve this interaction:

1.

2.

3.

4.

5.

6.

7.

8.

9.

10.

Learning Activity 1-1: Communication Basics

Over the course of your professional career as an OTA, you will have the opportunity to meet and work with many clients in occupational therapy. It is useful to practice some standard opening lines ahead of time to help you display confidence and make a positive first impression. In the space below, write several sentences you might use initially when introducing yourself to a new client, such as Susan Smythe, a 70-year-old female who had total hip replacement surgery 2 days ago.

OTA introduction:

Now check your introductory statement against the following suggestions in this chapter to determine if all the necessary elements are present.

For an initial encounter with an adult client, it is more respectful for an OTA to use an appropriate title such as "Mr." or "Mrs." and the client's last name. Ensure you are pronouncing the person's name correctly. For the above client, Susan Smythe, her last name could be pronounced either with a short or long "i" sound in the middle. It is courteous to ascertain which pronunciation is correct. Next, tell the client your name and discipline. It is important to realize that an OTA should be referred to as an "occupational therapy practitioner" or "occupational therapy assistant" and not as a "therapist" (American Occupational Therapy Association [AOTA], 2009, 2010b; Centers for Medicare & Medicaid Services [CMS], 2008, 2012). Also acknowledge your working relationship with the client's occupational therapist (OT) and/or physician who referred the client to occupational therapy. The OTA might also determine if the client has an understanding of occupational therapy and/or ask how the client is feeling. Of course, each client encounter will be a little different depending on the circumstances. Here are some examples of introductory statements that an OTA might use with a client recovering from hip surgery:

- *Hello Mrs. Smythe, I am Valerie Veracity, an occupational therapy assistant student. Am I saying your last name correctly? It is very nice to meet you. I have been working with your occupational therapist, Karen, and she asked me to see you today to review your hip precautions and teach you how to manage putting on your socks and shoes. How are you feeling today?*

- *Good morning, Mrs. Smythe. My name is Valerie Veracity and I am from the occupational therapy department. Dr. Smith ordered occupational therapy to help you recover from your hip surgery. I am an occupational therapy assistant student working with Karen Karing, the therapist who evaluated you yesterday. Would you like me to explain further what occupational therapy is?*

- *Hello Mrs. Smythe. I am Sally Smiley, an occupational therapy assistant. Am I pronouncing your last name correctly? Your occupational therapist, Karen, asked me to work with you today to teach you how to get dressed without bending your hip. How does your hip feel today?*

- *Hello Mrs. Smythe. I am Sally Smiley, an occupational therapy assistant. Am I saying your last name correctly? Your surgeon referred you to occupational therapy so we can teach you how to manage safely at home with your hip precautions. I work closely with Karen Karing, your occupational therapist, and Karen asked me to see you today. Do you have any questions before we start?*

- *Good morning, Mrs. Smythe, it is nice to meet you. I am Sally Smiley, your occupational therapy practitioner for today. Karen, the occupational therapist whom you have been working with this week, asked me to teach you how to get dressed safely with your hip precautions. Do you remember what equipment Karen gave you yesterday to help you dress?*

Now write an introduction you might use for John Valorie, whom you are meeting for the first time. He had a below-knee amputation 5 days ago and was evaluated by the OT yesterday.

Learning Activity 1-2: What Is Occupational Therapy?

Some people are not aware of occupational therapy or may not fully understand the profession. The OT will typically explain what occupational therapy is during the initial client contact or evaluation. However, while coping with an illness, injury, or other circumstances, clients and families/significant others usually encounter multiple health team members and are often overwhelmed, confused, or tired. As a result, the distinct value of occupational therapy may remain unclear to them at this time. Thus, the OTA must be ready to provide a clear and simple definition of occupational therapy appropriate to the client's situation, and explain briefly how that client will benefit. The AOTA website (www.aota.org) and official documents, such as *The Philosophical Base of Occupational Therapy* (AOTA, 2011) and *Occupational Therapy Practice Framework: Domain and Process* (AOTA, 2014), are useful resources to help you define occupational therapy for different audiences. Also, Table 1-1 presents practical suggestions for communicating with clients and others effectively.

Create a brief definition of occupational therapy that you might use with clients or family/caregivers.

Occupational therapy is...

Now develop a brief definition that you might use to explain occupational therapy to other professionals or service providers (i.e., medical interns, teachers, school administrators, optometrists, etc.).

Occupational therapy is...

Table 1-1
Suggestions for Initial Client Encounters and Occupational Therapy Definition

Do

- Make a sincere effort to have eye contact with the person you are addressing, particularly if you must review paperwork, jot down notations, or enter information on the computer during the encounter.
- Pay close attention to what the person is saying or doing.
- Use simple, easy-to-understand language.
- Make your definition brief and uncomplicated.
- Explain what "occupation" means.
- Relate to the individual client's condition, situation, or problem.
- Discuss how occupational therapy can help.
- Differentiate occupational therapy from other disciplines.
- Consider what is appropriate for that practice setting, time frames, and reasonable for the client's circumstances.
- Clarify the focus of your intervention for that particular client relating to occupation, such as enabling independence, remediating particular client factors to improve function, facilitating skills or occupational adaptations, assessing safety, providing caregiver education, modifying the environment, and improving comfort or quality of life.
- Provide examples or describe briefly the use of preparatory tasks and methods, therapeutic activities and occupations, adaptive equipment, or other specialized interventions indicated for this client.

Don't

- Do not appear preoccupied with other matters, such as personal problems, casual conversations with staff, or paperwork.
- Do not use technical jargon or abbreviations (unless you explain them). Clients may not know what ADL, COTA, OTR, CVA, etc., stand for, or the meaning of words such as "activities of daily living," "dysphagia," "sensory integration," or "myocardial infarction."
- Do not talk down to the client or act as if the client is unintelligent.
- Do not refer to an adult client with nicknames such as "honey" or "sweetie."
- Do not refer to an OTA as a "therapist."
- Do not use an identical explanation for each client. Not all clients will achieve complete independence or improved functional abilities, as some conditions are irreversible or terminal. However, occupational therapy can help clients maintain function and manage chronic conditions for improved quality of life. The focus of occupational therapy interventions may be different according to various circumstances, but will contribute to occupational performance in some way.
- Do not guarantee results, but instead explain areas that will be addressed or may realistically improve based on sound clinical knowledge.
- Do not overwhelm the client with too much information.
- Do not ask the client a question you really do not want an answer to. For example, if you say, "Do you want to come to therapy today?" that sets up the client to refuse treatment. It might be better to say, "It is time for your occupational therapy session now." If you ask the client, "How was your day today?", be prepared to hear about bland hospital food, a noisy roommate, or how the television or phone did not work properly. You might decide it is better to target a question toward the client's condition, such as, "How does your hip feel today?"
- Do not lie, create false hope, or unrealistic expectations. However, how you temper the truth can have a significant effect in helping to prevent client hopelessness and despair.

Worksheet 1-2

It Looks Like You Play All Day

A group of physicians are taking a tour of the rehabilitation department. When they arrive at the occupational therapy clinic, the physicians observe the following client interventions happening:

- A 70-year-old female client baking cookies
- A 65-year-old male client stacking cones
- A 53-year-old female client putting pegs in a pegboard
- A 38-year-old female client standing and placing cans on a shelf
- A 22-year-old male client playing checkers with an OTA

One of the physicians comments, *"It looks like you must play with toys all day in here."* How might an OTA respond to this?

Learning Activity 1-3: Explaining Occupational Therapy's Role

For each of the following situations, role-play with a partner or write a brief paragraph below. Introduce yourself as an OTA or student and explain the unique role of occupational therapy for that client and general desired, realistic outcome. For this exercise, assume each client has been evaluated by the OT and is just beginning the first treatment session.

1. *Early intervention:* Mary Mackie is a single parent of 20-month-old Alexis. Alexis was recently diagnosed with a developmental disability; is nonverbal; has poor eye contact, oral-motor sensitivity, and tactile defensiveness; and does not walk yet.

2. *Outpatient clinic:* Jane Doe is a 40-year-old married bookkeeper with children ages 2 and 5. Jane sustained a Colle's fracture in her dominant upper extremity 6 weeks ago. The cast was removed last week and she has not returned to work yet. Her hand is swollen, painful, and stiff, causing difficulty with basic (BADL) and instrumental (IADL) activities of daily living.

3. *School setting:* Jack Springer is the parent of Steven, a second-grade student with a learning disability. Steven demonstrates poor handwriting, difficulty using scissors, poor time management, and decreased organizational skills. Steven's delayed skills acquisition creates difficulty with completing class assignments and managing clothing for gym and recess.

4. *Skilled nursing facility:* Karen Kairgiver is the adult child and health care agent of Ruth Rezzydent, a client with moderate dementia. Ruth has lived in a long-term care facility for the past year but fell out of bed last week, breaking her hip. She is 1-week status post total hip replacement surgery.

5. *Acute care hospital:* Mike O'Malley, a 75-year-old retired plumber, had a heart attack 5 days ago. He lives with his wife in a private house and was independent prior to his hospitalization.

6. *Rehabilitation hospital:* Marvin Billings is an 18-year-old male who sustained a C6 spinal cord injury due to a diving accident in his backyard.

7. *Inpatient behavioral health setting:* Judy Jones is a 21-year-old female diagnosed with a cocaine addiction. She lives at home with her parents, recently dropped out of college, and was arrested for drug possession a few days ago. She was admitted to an inpatient drug rehabilitation program in lieu of going to jail.

Worksheet 1-3

Do You Know What You Are Doing?

Your client, realizing you are a student or novice practitioner, may express concern about your knowledge base or ability to handle his or her situation. The client may state, *"Have you ever worked with someone like me before?"* or *"Do you know what you are doing?"*

How can you respond appropriately while being truthful about your limited experience?

Worksheet 1-4

Are You Really Sure You Can Do This?

Clients often experience anxiety and uncertainty regarding their health condition or circumstances. They may express various concerns regarding occupational therapy, other health team members, care received, or upcoming events. It is important that you respond appropriately to help put the client's mind at ease. Consider how you might respond to the following client scenarios, assuming that you are competent in the particular task at hand:

1. Your client is concerned about your ability to transfer him safely and states, *"I am a big guy and you are so tiny. I really don't think you can get me into that wheelchair."*

2. While performing a cooking task in occupational therapy, your client expresses fear regarding functional ambulation and states, *"I am afraid my weak leg will buckle and I will fall."*

3. As you are about to transfer a client from wheelchair to bed, your client states, *"I don't want you to get hurt moving me."*

Using Empathy

Tables 1-2 and 1-3 (Tufano, 1997) provide useful tips to help you develop therapeutic communication skills and acknowledge client feelings effectively. To practice empathetic responses, complete Worksheet 1-5, Worksheet 1-6, and Learning Activity 1-4.

Table 1-2
Guidelines to Help Form a Primary Accurate Empathy Response

- Attend fully to the client, especially to nonverbal clues. (Refer back to the section on attending and listening skills.)
- Identify the feelings expressed by the client in the present. Do not become distracted by focusing on the past. Even when your client is telling a story in the past tense, he or she is experiencing feelings in the present.
- Select the most dominant feeling expressed. Clients may experience more than one emotion at a time. Choose the one that is most evident.
- Match the correct intensity of feeling expressed. Think of feelings as having three levels—mild, moderate, and severe. For example, a mild form of the feeling word *anger* is upset, a moderate form is mad, and a severe form is rage. Practice identifying the levels of intensity on your own.
- Paraphrase the main idea associated with the client's experiences and behaviors. Stay close to the client's words, but deviate enough to let him or her know that you are listening.
- Formulate a verbal response consisting of "You feel _____ because _____."
- Check your empathic response for accuracy. After formulating your verbal response, ask the client what he or she thinks about your statement. Does he or she agree or disagree?

Reprinted with permission from Tufano, R. (1997). Therapeutic communication. In K. Sladyk (Ed.), *OT student primer: A guide to college success* (pp. 223-240). Thorofare, NJ: SLACK Incorporated.

Table 1-3
Guidelines of What to Avoid When Formulating an Emphatic Response

- Avoid not responding at all. Sometimes therapists lack a response because they are not sure how to phrase their statement. The client may interpret this lack of response as not caring or disinterest.
- Avoid asking a question when you should be conveying understanding. The client may interpret your question as a sign of inattentiveness and may think that his or her statement was not worth responding to.
- Avoid using clichés (e.g., Don't worry, be happy). You want to individualize your responses and support the uniqueness of each person.
- Avoid giving advice. During the early stages of developing a therapeutic relationship, it is not timely to jump into action. Take the time to listen and understand your client thoroughly. Many people want to be heard and are not interested in your solutions.
- Avoid pretending to understand when you genuinely do not. If you are genuinely confused, the appropriate skill to use is open questioning. Clients can tell whether you are trying to understand or just placating them.
- Avoid parroting the client's exact words. You want to avoid sounding mechanical or incapable of understanding.
- Avoid giving sympathy in place of empathy. Sympathy connotes identification with the client's feelings such as pity, condolence, compassion, and commiseration. It also suggests that you agree with your client's feelings. When you use empathy effectively, it does not matter whether you agree with the client or not. One does not have to agree to understand where the client is coming from.

Reprinted with permission from Tufano, R. (1997). Therapeutic communication. In K. Sladyk (Ed.), *OT student primer: A guide to college success* (pp. 223-240). Thorofare, NJ: SLACK Incorporated.

Worksheet 1-5

I Want to Walk

Consider the therapeutic communication techniques you might use when responding to the following situations.

1. You are working with Hector, a 22-year-old carpenter who recently sustained a C6 spinal cord injury due to a fall from a roof. As you are discussing his occupational therapy goals for the next few weeks, Hector tells you the doctors are wrong and his main goal is to walk again. You know this is unrealistic based on the medical reports. What would you say to him?

2. You are working with Melvin, a 68-year-old male with a total hip replacement. He has non-weight-bearing status for his affected lower extremity and is presently using a walker with moderate assistance. Today you are trying to teach Melvin how to don his socks and shoes using adaptive equipment. He tells you that the equipment is "silly," his wife can help him dress, and that his only goal is to walk again. What would you say to him?

Morreale, M. J. (2015). *Developing clinical competence: A workbook for the OTA*. Thorofare, NJ: SLACK Incorporated.

Worksheet 1-6

This Feels Like Kindergarten

Your client, Keith, is a 62-year-old defense attorney whose hobbies include gardening and woodworking. Keith has undergone surgery to repair a lacerated median nerve and is now at the strengthening phase in therapy. He has not returned to work yet due to hypersensitivity in his hand and difficulty grasping and manipulating objects. To implement the occupational therapy intervention plan, you place the client's affected hand in a plastic shoebox filled with uncooked rice and ask him to locate and remove small objects (i.e., blocks, beads) with the affected hand. The client seems offended and states, *"I feel like I am in kindergarten with my grandkids! My children would really laugh if they saw me, a pit-bull defense lawyer, doing this."*

How would you respond to those statements?

To address this client's specific deficits and likely goals, what activities and occupations could you choose that might be more meaningful for this client?

Morreale, M. J. (2015). *Developing clinical competence: A workbook for the OTA*. Thorofare, NJ: SLACK Incorporated.

Learning Activity 1-4: I Don't Want Therapy

Consider the therapeutic communication techniques you might use when responding to the following situations.

1. A client was admitted to an acute care hospital with an exacerbation of chronic obstructive pulmonary disease, and her anticipated discharge is in 3 days. The client was evaluated by the OT yesterday. Today you enter the client's hospital room in the morning and tell her it is time for occupational therapy. The client states, *"Please go away. I just did a lot of leg exercises and walking in PT (physical therapy). I am too tired for any more therapy."* What would you say to her?

2. Your client is 80 years old and diagnosed with rheumatoid arthritis. He has pain and stiffness in both upper extremities, causing difficulties with ADL. Today he arrives at the outpatient clinic accompanied by his wife who states, *"My husband doesn't need all this. He had therapy before and it did not help. I don't know why the doctor made us come here."* What would you say to them?

3. Your client in home care is a 67-year-old male who has terminal pancreatic cancer. During his occupational therapy session he states, *"What's the use of all this therapy? The doctor told me I only have 6 months to live. This is a complete waste of time."* What would you say to him?

Morreale, M. J. (2015). *Developing clinical competence: A workbook for the OTA*. Thorofare, NJ: SLACK Incorporated.

Learning Activity 1-5: I Don't Need a Job

Clients who are unfamiliar with occupational therapy often take the word *occupation* literally, erroneously believing the profession entails finding jobs for people. Consider how you might respond to the following situations.

1. A 22-year-old college student was admitted to the hospital 2 days ago with bilateral leg fractures and internal injuries due to a motor vehicle accident. He was evaluated by the OT yesterday. Today you enter the client's hospital room and tell him it is time for occupational therapy. The client states, *"I don't need a job now. What I need is to get out of here to finish up my bachelor's degree and go to law school in the fall."* How would you respond to those statements?

2. Your client is 78 years old and diagnosed with Parkinson's disease. He has decreased bilateral upper extremity range of motion and strength, along with a history of falling. Today he arrives at the outpatient clinic accompanied by his wife who states, *"My husband certainly doesn't need a job at his age. He hasn't worked in years! I don't know why the doctor made us come here."* How would you respond to those statements?

3. A toddler diagnosed with a developmental delay started receiving early intervention services only recently. Today the child's father took the day off from work to observe his daughter's therapy program. During the occupational therapy session the parent states, *"Do you always start training disabled kids this early for a job? My daughter is only 2! How do you know what she is going to want to be?"* How would you respond?

4. Your client is a 55-year-old plumber who recently had cardiac bypass surgery. During his occupational therapy session he states, *"What's the use of this job therapy? Forget about me getting a job. The doctor told me I won't be able to go back to work. This is all a waste of time."* How would you respond to those statements?

Worksheet 1-7
Asking Open-Ended Questions

Clients may express vague, disingenuous, or limited statements about their condition, circumstances, or emotional status. While closed questions are appropriate for situations requiring a very specific response (such as if a sensory stimulus can be felt or asking if the client is tired), open-ended questions help the OTA elicit further information to clarify the client's situation, perception, or emotions (Cole, 2012; Tufano, 1997). To avoid a simple "yes" or "no" response when asking a client questions, Tufano (1997) lists the following words as helpful sentence starters: where, how, why, when, what, tell, describe. Use caution with the word *why*, as that could be perceived as judgmental (Cole, 2012; Tufano, 1997). For each of the following client statements, develop several open-ended questions to obtain pertinent information from the client.

1. My shoulder hurts.

2. I can't do anything right.

3. I fell in my apartment.

4. My life is a charade.

5. I never thought I would turn out like this.

6. My hand is useless.

7. I'm so confused.

8. I lost my job.

9. I hate school.

10. I am no good in gym class.

Adapted from Tufano, R. (1997). Therapeutic communication. In K. Sladyk (Ed.), *OT student primer: A guide to college success* (pp. 223-240). Thorofare, NJ: SLACK Incorporated.

Worksheet 1-8

Eliciting Information Efficiently

Nick, an OTA, is meeting his client, Jean Jones, for the first time. Jean is a 60-year-old female recently hospitalized and diagnosed with Guillain-Barré syndrome. Yesterday Jean was transferred from acute care to a rehabilitation hospital and subsequently evaluated by the OT, Karen. Today the OT asked Nick to obtain further information about the client's living situation. Consider Nick and Jean's initial conversation below. What suggestions would you make regarding the OTA's interaction with the client?

OTA: Hello Jean, I am Nick, an occupational therapy assistant. It is very nice to meet you. Your occupational therapist, Karen, asked me to work with you today. Are you feeling better today?
Client: No.
OTA: Why do you say that?
Client: I'm terrible. Don't you know how weak I am? I can't do anything!
OTA: That's not true. When I came in I saw that you were doing a pretty good job feeding yourself with that device Karen gave you.
Client: Well, I spilled half of my food.
OTA: The nurses will be in soon to get you cleaned up. Anyway, can I ask you some questions?
Client: I would rather be left alone.
OTA: This won't take too long. Where do you reside?
Client: 1374 East Main Street—just a few blocks from here.
OTA: I mean, do you live in a house?
Client: No.
OTA: An apartment?
Client: No, a condo.
OTA: Do you have any stairs?
Client: Yes.
OTA: How many stairs?
Client: Do you mean inside or outside?
OTA: Both.
Client: Three steps outside and about 10 steps to the second floor.
OTA: OK, now tell me about your bathroom situation.
Client: Well, I occasionally get constipated so I have to drink a lot of prune juice.

Suggestions to improve this OTA's interaction with the client:

1.

2.

3.

4.

5.

Revise the interaction to incorporate more useful questions from the OTA:

Learning Activity 1-6: Active Listening

1. Think about a recent situation that took place in which you were not satisfied with the results. This could be with a roommate, coworker, friend, or teacher. Write down the specifics of the situation (i.e., dirty dishes always left in the sink; you always have to wash them; this makes you angry, etc.).

2. Next, write down what you remember you did or said. Include your tone of voice. Were you sitting or standing? How was your position in reference to the other person's? What were the other nonverbal signals you gave? What were those that you responded to from the other person?

3. Now, write down a new script. In this script, use "I" statements. Acknowledge the other person's situation, state the problem from your point of view, and suggest a solution. Think about possible responses that the other person might have, even role-play with a different person.

4. Now that you have thought through the communication barriers that originally took place, thought about a new way of approaching the issue, and role-played through it, try the real thing. Approach the individual, and try to communicate your concerns using your scripted version, remembering to keep "I" statements, reflect, and acknowledge the other person's feelings as well. I bet you work it out and feel better about the communication.

Reprinted with permission from Lowenstein, N., & Duncombe, L. (2002). Professional behaviors. In K. Sladyk (Ed.), *The successful occupational therapy fieldwork student* (pp. 23-32). Thorofare, NJ: SLACK Incorporated.

1. Situation:

2. Words and actions:

3. New script "I" statements:

4. New approach results:

Worksheet 1-9

Interaction OTA—Elementary School Student

Marisol is an entry-level OTA who works at an elementary school. Her client, Chrystal, is a second grade student with a developmental delay. Marisol and Chrystal had the following conversation during an intervention session. What suggestions would you make regarding the OTA's interaction with the student?

OTA: OK Chrystal, we are going to work some more on your handwriting today. Let's start with this worksheet.
Student: Do we have to?
OTA: Yes. You know your parents and teacher would like your work to be much neater. It will only get better if you practice.
Student: Writing is boring. Can't we do something else?
OTA: Not today. Would you like to choose a colored pencil from the box?
Student: No.
OTA: Chrystal, pick up a pencil. Any color you would like.
Student: Nope.
OTA: Don't be difficult. Please grab one of the pencils.
Student: What if I don't?
OTA: Well, you'll be sorry.
Student: What does that mean?
OTA: Do you want to see your parents again?
Student: Yes.
OTA: Well, you can't go home until you pick up a pencil and finish this worksheet.
Student: You can't make me stay here.
OTA: Oh yeah missy? I will tie you to the chair if I need to. Now pick up a pencil. Why are you crying now?
Student: You are yelling at me. I don't like that.
OTA: I am not yelling. I am just talking in a loud voice because you are being a bad girl. Come on now, start this worksheet. I will give you a sticker when you are finished.

Suggestions to improve this interaction:

1.

2.

3.

4.

5.

6.

7.

8.

Learning Activity 1-7: Nonverbal Communication

With a partner, choose a contemporary TV talk show (i.e., *The View, The Talk, The Five*, etc.) that has a panel of diverse hosts who discuss current events or controversial subjects. Watch the opening segment of the show with the sound off and observe how the talk show hosts interact with each other. Jot down the nonverbal behaviors you observed during the exchange and determine if you can ascertain the overall tone of the conversation. Can you tell which panelists seem to agree or disagree with the others? Did you and your partner interpret what you saw in the same way? What are the specific behaviors you and your partner each observed to reach your conclusions? After you complete this worksheet, watch the segment again—but with the sound on, so you can determine if your interpretation of nonverbal behaviors was correct.

Positive Nonverbal Behaviors Observed	*Negative Nonverbal Behaviors Observed*

- If you felt the panel's tone was congenial, did you observe any panelists smiling, nodding, hugging, lightly touching each other affectionately, or waiting to speak one's turn?

- If you felt the tone was aggressive or argumentative, did you observe panelists standing up, pointing, or exhibiting "in your face" behavior? Were people speaking over each other at the same time? What facial expressions did you observe? What behaviors indicated that people may have been shouting?

- Did any of the panelists "tune out" by looking away or moving elsewhere, crossing arms, sighing, or not actively participating?

Morreale, M. J. (2015). *Developing clinical competence: A workbook for the OTA*. Thorofare, NJ: SLACK Incorporated.

Learning Activity 1-8: Communication Styles

Watch a one-on-one TV interview performed by a celebrity interviewer who is perceived to have a more gentle or empathetic approach (such as Barbara Walters or Oprah Winfrey). Also watch an episode of a show where real people are interrogated by someone with a more direct style or tougher reputation (such as Dr. Phil or Judge Judy). Compare and contrast the two styles of questioning and the nonverbal behavior of the interviewers. Consider the following as you are watching the two interviews:

- What did the interviewers do or say to elicit the information they were trying to obtain?

- What specific open- or closed-ended questions did they ask?

- What tone of voice did the interviewers use?

- Were the styles of both interviewers equally effective?

- How did the persons being questioned respond verbally and nonverbally? Did they appear comfortable or uncomfortable?

- Was information freely shared or were responses vague and resistant?

- Do you feel any of the interviewers' questions or behaviors were inappropriate? Why or why not?

- Which interviewer appeared more sympathetic to an individual's situation, and why?

- Did an interviewer specifically acknowledge or guess at what the person was feeling? If so, was the interviewer's interpretation correct?

- What judgmental or empathetic words were used by the interviewers?

- How was active listening evident?

- Was either of the interviewer's approaches too soft or too tough?

- Which approach do you like better and why?

Answers to Worksheets

Worksheet 1-1: Initial Client Encounter

1. It is more respectful to call the elderly client "Mrs. Doe" rather than her first name.

2. *"Hey"* in the opening statement is not very professional. "Hello" or "Good morning" is more appropriate in this situation. Use appropriate language for the particular context and geographical area.

3. It is incorrect and unethical for the OTA to refer to herself as a *"therapist."* The OTA should use the terms *occupational therapy practitioner* or *occupational therapy assistant* instead (AOTA, 2009, 2010b; CMS, 2008, 2012).

4. As the question *"Any problems?"* is quite vague, the client responds about issues unrelated to her diagnosis.

5. The OTA uses unfamiliar abbreviations, such as OTA, which the client is not familiar with.

6. The OTA does not acknowledge her working relationship with the OT or physician, or mention that Jane was evaluated by the OT.

7. The purpose of the session, *"help you get dressed,"* does not reflect skilled therapy, as an aide or family member could help the client dress.

8. The OTA does not adequately explain what occupational therapy is, such as the meaning of "occupation" or goals of improving the client's function. There also needs to be a better distinction between the disciplines of occupational therapy and physical therapy.

9. Calling an adult client *"sweetie"* is disrespectful.

10. The OTA did not acknowledge the client's complaints.

Worksheet 1-2: It Looks Like You Play All Day

You might explain how occupational therapy practitioners use everyday objects to work on remediating different client factors and skills to improve a client's performance in daily living skills (occupations). Without breaching client confidentiality, you might relate the use of cones and pegs to improve specific motor function, such as elbow range of motion, cylindrical grip, or tip pinch, or to other essential skills, such as crossing midline. Cooking activities or checkers might be used to address specific cognitive/perceptual deficits, such as unilateral neglect or problems in sequencing, problem solving, or spatial relations. Standing and putting weighted cans on a shelf may help to restore balance, range of motion, strength, and endurance, which are all necessary for ADL performance. ***However, the occupational therapy department might internally use this experience to reflect upon whether enough occupation-based interventions are being implemented.***

Worksheet 1-3: Do You Know What You Are Doing?

In clinical practice, if you are expected to do a task you are very unsure of, you should discuss this with your supervisor (AOTA, 2009). It is unethical to perform interventions for which you are not competent (AOTA, 2010a, 2010b). Assuming you are competent with a particular client task, your communicative style should convey confidence in your abilities and professionalism. However, an OTA student or practitioner should never exaggerate or fabricate information about one's credentials or experience (AOTA, 2010a). As an OTA student, you might explain to the client that you have professional education in this area, are closely supervised, and would not do anything that would knowingly put the client in danger. As a novice OTA, you might add that you have fieldwork experience, have passed a national certification exam, and are licensed. If the client still appears concerned, you might ask another colleague or your supervisor to oversee or assist with the task.

Worksheet 1-4: Are You Really Sure You Can Do This?

For these kinds of situations it is imperative that the client feel safe and that you demonstrate understanding of the client's concerns, such as fear of falling or getting hurt. Your demeanor and communication should convey confidence and professionalism, but you have an ethical obligation to only attempt tasks that are you are competent to perform (AOTA, 2010a, 2010b). You might convey your professional education, practice, and experience. Reassure the client that you would not do anything that would be unsafe. Explain the procedure and address the client's specific concerns such as, *"I will support your knee with my leg so it can't buckle"* or *"I have transferred a lot of people much bigger than you and will not let you fall. This transfer belt will ensure that you will be safe."* If the client still appears concerned, you might ask another colleague or your supervisor to stand by or assist with the task. Sometimes humor can even be an effective method with select clients such as, *"I am a lot stronger than I look—this lab coat is hiding my huge muscles!"*

Worksheet 1-5: I Want to Walk

1. Sometimes clients have great difficulty accepting the reality of a situation. They may be scared, confused, angry, or in denial. You might acknowledge and validate the client's feelings, but without giving false hope. Tufano (1997) provides useful tips for therapeutic communication such as respect, genuineness, attending, effective listening, asking open questions, and using primary accurate empathy. The following useful formula is suggested for occupational therapy practitioners to show empathy and understand feelings:

    "You feel ___ because _____ " (Cole 2012, p. 74; Tufano, 1997, p. 234).

    You might say, *"You feel angry and overwhelmed because this is a huge life-changing event and you don't know how you will be able to cope. Is that correct?"* However, it is a balancing act to gently acknowledge the truth while not causing hopelessness and despair. During the exchange you might say, *"You had a very, very serious injury. We need to first focus on achieving your other goals during the next few weeks like being able to feed yourself and operating a wheelchair"* or *"I am so sorry that your injury is not likely to make walking a feasible goal. However, we are all here to help you become as independent as possible. I can tell that you are very determined and will be able to manage many things on your own."* Of course, you may encourage the client to continue to express his feelings and to attend support groups and counseling as appropriate.

2. It is important to reinforce how the client can benefit from occupational therapy. The intervention plan should include client-centered goals that the OTA can reinforce with the client. You can acknowledge the client's frustration, *"You feel frustrated because you have to go through all this effort when you just want to be up and about."* You might then go on to say, *"Tomorrow we will be working on arm exercises so you can have enough strength and endurance to manage using your walker at home"* or *"The doctor said you are not allowed to bend for several months because of your surgery. This equipment will allow you to be independent again at home, like you were before your surgery. I am sure your wife would appreciate that."*

Worksheet 1-6: This Feels Like Kindergarten

If a client seems offended performing a preparatory task that is otherwise not normally age appropriate, you might say something like, *"It sounds like you might be feeling a bit insulted doing this. I'm sorry—that is not my intent."* Acknowledge that, although the activity might appear "juvenile" on the surface, there is indeed a specific therapeutic purpose. When implementing preparatory interventions, you should make it a point to relate the task to the particular client factors and performance skills you are remediating, and also explain how this relates to occupational performance. In this case, the task was chosen to help reduce hypersensitivity and improve manipulation skills of the affected hand to enable occupations such as writing, using a computer keyboard, and performing hobbies. ***Better yet, incorporate activities and occupations into the client's treatment program whenever possible.*** Rather than presenting this client with the aforementioned preparatory task that offended him, this client may have benefited more from a "real-life" task such as handling soil for a gardening activity, using a sanding block to sand wood, or utilizing a built-up pen for writing.

Worksheet 1-7: Asking Open-Ended Questions

Here are some suggestions, although you may come up with other questions.

1. My shoulder hurts.
    o *Describe your shoulder pain—or—What does your shoulder pain feel like?*
    o *What makes your shoulder pain better or worse?*
    o *How does the pain affect your daily activities?*
    o *When does the pain occur?*

2. I can't do anything right.
    o *What do you mean by that?*
    o *How long have you felt this way?*
    o *Describe a situation that causes you to feel that way.*
    o *What would you like to change?*

3. I fell in my apartment.
   o *How did you fall in your apartment?*
   o *What happened after you fell?*
   o *How long ago did you fall in your apartment?*
   o *What might you have done differently to prevent falling?*
4. My life is a charade.
   o *What do you mean by that statement?*
   o *How is your life a charade?*
   o *What are your plans for the future?*
   o *What are some things you wish you had done differently?*
5. I never thought I would turn out like this.
   o *How do you see yourself?*
   o *How do you feel about… (i.e., your arrest, addiction to cocaine, homelessness, etc.)?*
   o *How do you think you could turn things around?*
   o *What are your goals?*
   o *What would you like to change?*
6. My hand is useless.
   o *What specific problems are you having with your hand?*
   o *When did you start having difficulty with your hand?*
   o *How does your hand condition affect your daily activities?*
   o *What types of things are hard to do with your hand?*
7. I'm so confused.
   o *What things are confusing you?*
   o *What else are you feeling?*
   o *What would help you to understand?*
   o *How can you get more information?*
8. I lost my job.
   o *What are your plans?*
   o *How does that affect you and your family?*
   o *What happened that caused you to lose your job?*
   o *What might have happened differently to avoid getting fired?*
9. I hate school.
   o *What do you hate about school?*
   o *What would you like to change about school?*
   o *Describe what makes you feel that way about school.*
   o *How long have you felt this way?*
10. I am no good in gym class.
    o *What specific things in gym class are hard for you?*
    o *Tell me how that makes you feel.*
    o *What would you like to be better at?*
    o *What are some things you feel you are good at in school?*

Worksheet 1-8: Eliciting Information Efficiently

Clearly, in this scenario, the OTA is not using appropriate open-ended questions to elicit the desired information in a timely manner. Cole (2012, p. 74) suggests that in order to prevent a simple yes or no response, the OT should avoid the following as question starters: "do you, can you, would you, are you, and have you." Here are some additional suggestions for improving this client interaction:

1. It is more respectful to call the client Mrs. Jones rather than Jean.
2. The OTA should explain the purpose of the session.
3. The OTA should demonstrate empathy and address her concerns when the client reports feeling "terrible" or when the client expresses frustration regarding spilling her food.
4. The OTA should acknowledge that the client has particular feelings, but instead he insinuates that Mrs. Jones should not feel that way.
5. The OTA should use open- rather than closed-ended questions.
6. The OTA needs to phrase questions more clearly to target the desired information in a concise manner.

Here is the same exchange in a more useful format:

OTA: Hello Mrs. Jones, I am Nick, an occupational therapy assistant. It is very nice to meet you. Your occupational therapist, Karen, asked me to work with you today to discuss your living situation so we can start planning how you will manage at home. How are you today?
Client: Terrible.
OTA: What is making you feel terrible?
Client: Don't you know how weak I am? I can't do anything!
OTA: You are feeling very frustrated because your illness is making everything more difficult for you. Is that correct? [Client nods her head yes.] However, I can tell by the way you were just feeding yourself that you are a very determined person. I am sure you will make a lot of progress here.
Client: Do you really think so?
OTA: Absolutely. Now please tell me about your living situation—what type of place do you live in and who might be around to help?
Client: I live with my husband in a condo. My daughter lives a few miles away and I have a good friend who lives next door to me.
OTA: That's great. I would like to know more about the physical layout of your condo, such as the number of steps and how the bathroom is situated.
Client: I have three steps outside and about 10 steps to the second floor. There is a powder room on the first level and a full bathroom on the second level, next to my bedroom.

The OTA would continue interviewing the client in this manner until all the desired information is obtained.

Worksheet 1-9: Interaction OTA—Elementary School Student

1. Schools strive to create a welcoming and safe environment for students. Policies are created to prevent harassment, intimidation, and bullying (HIB) of students and a variety of resources are available (New Jersey Department of Education, 2010; Ohio Department of Education, 2014). This OTA is intimidating the student with language that is unacceptable. Scaring the student by threatening, "I will tie you to the chair" and "I will not let you see you parents" may cause emotional harm to the student. The OTA's behavior is clearly unprofessional and may result in severe disciplinary action.
2. The OTA is not maintaining professional composure as she is yelling at the student.
3. Do not ask a client if he or she "wants" to do a task if the answer "no" would be unacceptable.
4. It may be better to offer a specific choice to the student such as, "What color pencil do you want to use today—the red or green one?" or "Choose one of these two worksheets to work on today."
5. It might be better for the OTA to present the activity more positively, such as, "Let's show your parents how much better you are doing with your handwriting" or "We are going to do this worksheet in pretty rainbow colors. You can use a different colored pencil for each line."

6. By using appropriate verbal and nonverbal communication, the OTA must "set the tone" that he or she is an authority figure that deserves respect. However, it is not productive or professional to lose one's temper, yell, or get into an argument with a student.

7. Do not call a student "bad." It is the child's specific behavior and language that are unacceptable. The OTA might say, "You are talking back to me and not following directions. That is not acceptable."

8. Use therapeutic communication techniques such as therapeutic use of self, behavior modification, or even making the activity into a "game." Here are some examples:

"If you form all the letters correctly today, I will give you a special prize today."

or

"If you can finish this worksheet before the timer goes off, I will give you an extra sticker."

or

"After you finish this worksheet, I will put it on my bulletin board because I am proud of how hard you have been working on your handwriting this month."

or

"You feel writing is boring because it is not easy for you and you don't like to practice—is that right? I understand. Let's just work on this for 10 minutes and then we will do something fun."

References

American Occupational Therapy Association. (2009). Guidelines for supervision, roles, and responsibilities during the delivery of occupational therapy services. *American Journal of Occupational Therapy, 63*(6), 797-803. doi: 10.5014/ajot.63.6.797

American Occupational Therapy Association. (2010a). Occupational therapy code of ethics and ethics standards (2010). *American Journal of Occupational Therapy, 64*(6 Suppl.), S17-S26. doi: 10.5014/ajot.2010.64S17

American Occupational Therapy Association. (2010b). Standards of practice for occupational therapy. *American Journal of Occupational Therapy, 64*(6 Suppl.), S106-S111. doi: 10.5014/ajot.2010.64S106

American Occupational Therapy Association. (2011). The philosophical base of occupational therapy. *American Journal of Occupational Therapy, 65*(6 Suppl.), S65. doi:10.5014/ajot.2011.65S65

American Occupational Therapy Association. (2014). Occupational therapy practice framework: Domain and process (3rd ed.). *American Journal of Occupational Therapy, 68*(1 Suppl.), S1-S48. doi: 10.5014/ajot.2014.682006

Centers for Medicare & Medicaid Services. (2008). *Medicare Benefit Policy Manual* (Pub. 100-02: Ch. 15, Section 230.2). Baltimore, MD: Centers for Medicare & Medicaid Services. Retrieved from www.cms.gov/Regulations-and-Guidance/Guidance/Manuals/Downloads/bp102c15.pdf

Centers for Medicare & Medicaid Services. (2012). *Medicare Benefit Policy Manual* (Pub. 100-02: Ch. 15, Section 220). Baltimore, MD: Centers for Medicare & Medicaid Services. Retrieved from www.cms.gov/Regulations-and-Guidance/Guidance/Manuals/Downloads/bp102c15.pdf

Cole, M. (2012). *Group dynamics in occupational therapy: The theoretical basis and practice application of group intervention* (4th ed.). Thorofare, NJ: SLACK Incorporated.

Lowenstein, N., & Duncombe, L. (2002). Professional behaviors. In K. Sladyk (Ed.), *The successful occupational therapy fieldwork student* (pp. 23-32). Thorofare, NJ: SLACK Incorporated.

New Jersey Department of Education. (2010). *Harassment, intimidation, & bullying (HIB)*. Retrieved from www.state.nj.us/education/students/safety/behavior/hib/

Ohio Department of Education. (2014). *Anti-harassment, intimidation and bullying resources*. Retrieved from http://education.ohio.gov/Topics/Other-Resources/School-Safety/Safe-and-Supportive-Learning/Anti-Harassment-Intimidation-and-Bullying-Resource

Tufano, R. (1997). Therapeutic communication. In K. Sladyk (Ed.), *OT student primer: A guide to college success* (pp. 223-240). Thorofare, NJ: SLACK Incorporated.

Chapter 2

Demonstrating Professionalism

Professional behaviors for occupational therapy practitioners include traits such as dependability, punctuality, a well-groomed appearance, and appropriate demeanor. OTs and OTAs must also meet professional standards for attire, workplace conduct, and oral and written communication, plus demonstrate ethical behavior, good time management, and organizational skills. This chapter presents worksheets and learning activities to help you develop professional behaviors and skills necessary for fieldwork and clinical practice. Suggested answers to worksheets are provided at the end of the chapter.

Contents

Morreale, M. J.
Developing Clinical Competence: A Workbook for the OTA (pp. 29-67).
© 2015 SLACK Incorporated.

Worksheet 2-1

Scheduling Fieldwork

Always follow your academic fieldwork coordinator's specific instructions regarding the scheduling of fieldwork, such as if you should contact your fieldwork educator by phone or email.

For this exercise, consider the following information when answering the first two questions.
You have just been assigned Level I fieldwork for the spring semester. Your academic fieldwork coordinator provided the facility name and address, name of your fieldwork educator, a contact phone number, and an email address. You must contact the site directly to schedule your fieldwork. The fieldwork consists of 3 full days, which do not have to be consecutive but must be completed by May 15th. It is now February 1st.

1. You would really like to complete your fieldwork during Spring Break (the third week of April) when you do not have classes. When should you first attempt to contact the fieldwork site to set up your fieldwork dates?
   A. One week before you plan on completing the fieldwork
   B. One month before you plan on completing the fieldwork
   C. Beginning of February
   D. Beginning of March
   E. Beginning of April

2. You called your fieldwork site as directed, but your fieldwork educator was not available at that time. You left a message with the department secretary asking the fieldwork educator to call you back. It is 2 days later and you have still not heard back. Which of the following is your best course of action?
   A. Contact your academic fieldwork coordinator
   B. Wait another day or two for the fieldwork educator to call back
   C. Wait another week for the fieldwork educator to call back
   D. Call again and leave another message if your fieldwork educator is again unavailable
   E. Call again and ask to speak with the rehabilitation director if your fieldwork educator is still unavailable

3. You contact your fieldwork educator by phone, and this person informs you that you are assigned a different fieldwork educator at that site. Which of the following is your best course of action?
   A. Thank the person and state that you will need to cancel the fieldwork
   B. Thank the person but afterward ask your academic fieldwork coordinator for a new fieldwork site
   C. Ask to speak with that new fieldwork educator and notify your academic fieldwork coordinator of the change
   D. Tell the person on the phone that the change is not acceptable because you need to complete the fieldwork exactly as it was assigned to you
   E. Ask to speak with the rehabilitation director

Morreale, M. J. (2015). *Developing clinical competence: A workbook for the OTA*. Thorofare, NJ: SLACK Incorporated.

Worksheet 2-1 (continued)

Scheduling Fieldwork

4. You contacted your fieldwork educator several weeks ago to schedule your Level I fieldwork. The fieldwork is supposed to begin tomorrow, but you just became ill with a bad stomach virus that is causing severe nausea and diarrhea. Which of the following is your best course of action?

    A. Contact the site immediately to inform your fieldwork educator that you are ill and must reschedule the fieldwork

    B. Take some medicine, get a good night's sleep, and attend fieldwork even if you still are having symptoms

    C. Contact your academic fieldwork coordinator and ask that person to notify the site about your pending absence tomorrow

    D. Ask a family member or friend to call the site and notify your fieldwork educator about your pending absence tomorrow

    E. Bring a doctor's note to fieldwork tomorrow to prove your illness and ask your fieldwork educator if you have to stay or not

5. A week before you are to begin Level II fieldwork, your fieldwork educator calls to inform you that, due to several staff members on sick leave, your fieldwork must be rescheduled to 1 month later than you were originally scheduled to begin. This will conflict with your next Level II fieldwork. Which of the following is your best course of action?

    A. Thank the person for calling but state that you must cancel fieldwork at that site

    B. Thank the person for calling but state you will need to discuss this with your academic fieldwork coordinator

    C. Let the fieldwork educator know this will inconvenience you greatly and indicate it is unfair this happened so close to your scheduled starting date

    D. Insist strongly that you must complete the fieldwork during the exact dates that were assigned to you

    E. Ask to speak with the rehabilitation director

6. You contact your fieldwork educator, Carrie Capable, by email. Carrie sends the following reply, *"Dear Student, I am sorry but the rehabilitation director has already assigned another fieldwork student to me at this time. However, I have forwarded your message to Ellen Ethical, OTR, as she will be your supervisor instead. She will contact you by email today or tomorrow."* Which of the following is your best course of action?

    A. Send an email to the rehabilitation director regarding this situation

    B. Reply by email to thank Carrie Capable but also state that you will need to cancel the fieldwork

    C. Reply by email to thank Carrie Capable and then wait several days for the new fieldwork educator to contact you

    D. Call the fieldwork site and ask to speak with Ellen Ethical today as you do not have her email address

    E. Reply by email and ask Carrie Capable if it is possible for her to switch students

Worksheet 2-1 (continued)

Scheduling Fieldwork

7. As directed, you send an email to your fieldwork educator to set up your Level I fieldwork. It is 1 week later and you have not gotten any reply. Which of the following is your best course of action?

    A. Resend the original email to your fieldwork educator at this time

    B. Wait several more days for the fieldwork educator to reply

    C. Send another email to the fieldwork educator asking why that person has not replied and if there is a problem with the fieldwork

    D. Send an email to the rehabilitation director and copy the fieldwork educator and your academic fieldwork coordinator on the email

    E. Send an email to your academic fieldwork coordinator asking for assistance

8. You contacted your fieldwork educator several weeks ago to schedule your Level I fieldwork. The fieldwork is supposed to begin tomorrow but the weather forecast calls for some snow. You are nervous about driving in bad weather. Which of the following is your best course of action?

    A. Contact the site immediately to inform your fieldwork educator that you are not able to attend fieldwork tomorrow

    B. Get a good night's sleep, and check the weather forecast in the morning to decide if you will attend fieldwork or not

    C. Request that your academic fieldwork coordinator notify the site about your pending absence tomorrow

    D. Follow your college's policy regarding fieldwork absences

    E. Have your parent or guardian call to inform the fieldwork educator that you are not allowed to drive in bad weather

9. You are supposed to begin Level I fieldwork today at 8:30 a.m. However, you are stuck in traffic and will not be arriving until about 9:15 a.m. Which of the following is your best course of action?

    A. Once you arrive late, apologize profusely and promise it will not happen again

    B. Only when it is safe to do so, attempt to call, text, or email your clinical educator to notify the person of your impending lateness

    C. Turn around to return home and reschedule fieldwork for another day

    D. When you arrive at fieldwork, act as if nothing happened and hope that no one notices that you were late

    E. Once you arrive late, tell the fieldwork educator it really wasn't your fault that you were late and complain about all the traffic you encountered

10. Your Level I fieldwork is scheduled to begin tomorrow. However, your fieldwork educator contacts you today to inform you she needs to take the day off and must reschedule fieldwork to the following week. This change will cause you to be late handing in your fieldwork paper and timesheet to the academic fieldwork coordinator. Which of the following is your best course of action?

    A. Tell the fieldwork educator that this is not fair as you scheduled the fieldwork way ahead of time and you will now get a bad grade in class

    B. Firmly insist that you be assigned to another person tomorrow so you can complete the fieldwork on time

    C. Once the conversation is completed, hang up and then call your fieldwork educator's supervisor

    D. Reschedule fieldwork and contact your academic fieldwork coordinator to explain the situation

    E. Start crying and hope the fieldwork educator will do something to help you

Worksheet 2-2

Fieldwork Phone Interview

You must call your fieldwork educator as directed to set up your Level I fieldwork schedule. You have never been to this facility before and are not very familiar with the area. For each of the items below, indicate with a Y (yes) or N (no) if it is an appropriate topic for you to ask during the initial phone contact.

1. _____ Directions to the fieldwork site

2. _____ Start and end times for the day

3. _____ Where to meet in the facility

4. _____ If the facility is in a "bad" area

5. _____ Date(s) to complete fieldwork

6. _____ Amount of time for lunch

7. _____ Permission to come in late because you have to drive your kids to school

8. _____ If a lab coat is required

9. _____ Wearing of sneakers

10. _____ Availability of coffee or tea in the morning

11. _____ Permission to use your cell phone so you can monitor your children

12. _____ Permission to come in late or leave early to accommodate your bus or train schedule

13. _____ Permission to leave early to pick your children up from school

14. _____ Permission to leave early due to a dental appointment to get your teeth cleaned

15. _____ Permission to wear a head covering if required by your religion

16. _____ What paperwork to bring

17. _____ If it will be a very hard fieldwork, because a classmate failed fieldwork there last semester

18. _____ Reimbursement for gas and tolls

19. _____ If the fieldwork will require a lot of homework

20. _____ Types of diagnoses you will observe

Morreale, M. J. (2015). *Developing clinical competence: A workbook for the OTA*. Thorofare, NJ: SLACK Incorporated.

Worksheet 2-3

Directions to Fieldwork Site

List five ways to obtain directions to your fieldwork site without asking your fieldwork educator.

1.

2.

3.

4.

5.

Morreale, M. J. (2015). *Developing clinical competence: A workbook for the OTA.* Thorofare, NJ: SLACK Incorporated.

Worksheet 2-4

Dependability and Punctuality

Your fieldwork is scheduled to begin next week. List at least 10 things you can do to help ensure that you will get to fieldwork on time on your first day.

1.

2.

3.

4.

5.

6.

7.

8.

9.

10.

Morreale, M. J. (2015). *Developing clinical competence: A workbook for the OTA*. Thorofare, NJ: SLACK Incorporated.

Worksheet 2-5

Fieldwork Attire

Imagine you have been assigned fieldwork at an inpatient medical setting. You contacted your fieldwork educator and this person indicated that your client interventions will primarily consist of self-care occupations, transfers, and therapeutic exercises. Your fieldwork educator also informed you that the dress code is "business casual with a lab coat." For each of the items listed below, indicate with a Y (yes) or N (no) whether it is an appropriate choice for a fieldwork student to wear at this site. Explain why you chose each of your answers in the blank following the item.

1. _____ Scrubs_____

2. _____ Sneakers _____

3. _____ Flat, closed-toe shoes with rubber sole _____

4. _____ Dressy flip-flops _____

5. _____ Low-heeled leather sandals _____

6. _____ Heavy perfume/cologne/after shave _____

7. _____ Stud earrings _____

8. _____ Eyebrow piercing _____

9. _____ Head covering _____

10. _____ Visible underwear above pants waistband _____

11. _____ Neatly pressed dark jeans _____

12. _____ Khaki pants and a polo shirt _____

13. _____ Plain black sweatpants_____

14. _____ Sport tee shirt/jersey _____

15. _____ Button-down oxford shirt _____

16. _____ Dress slacks _____

17. _____ Cargo pants _____

18. _____ Polo shirt with collar and small designer logo emblem _____

19. _____ 32-inch plain gold necklace _____

20. _____ Charm bracelet _____

21. _____ Well-groomed, long artificial nails without polish _____

Morreale, M. J. (2015). *Developing clinical competence: A workbook for the OTA.* Thorofare, NJ: SLACK Incorporated.

Worksheet 2-5 (continued)

Fieldwork Attire

22. _____ Dark grey suit _____

23. _____ Name tag _____

24. _____ Solid color leggings _____

25. _____ Solid color hoodie _____

Learning Activity 2-1: Presentation and Demeanor

This next exercise, developed by Kasar and Clark (2000), helps participants improve awareness of how one is perceived and how one judges others based on appearance and behavior. It is a useful tool to facilitate understanding of the direct effects of one's demeanor, language, posture, and presentation and to explore how prior attitudes and values affect professionalism (Kasar & Clark, 2000). The steps for completing the activity are as follows:

Process

1. The instructor distributes worksheets.
2. Participants instructed to look about the room, observe other participants. Participants may walk about but refrain from talking.
3. Participants encouraged to observe body language, clothing, hairstyles, or any feature that would form an opinion.
4. Participants encouraged to make note of a previous event in their life that caused them to formulate a certain opinion/judgment/belief about the participant they are observing.
5. After 30 minutes observing time, instructor begins to encourage participants to disclose their observations and the reasons for their observations/opinions.
6. The worksheets have been constructed to elicit positive characteristics. However, the instructor should be sensitive to certain observations that may emerge and be prepared to handle comments that some of the participants may find discouraging/offensive.

Judging a Book by the Cover

1. Find someone who looks like they enjoy children.
   A. Reason:

2. Find someone who looks like they play sports.
   A. Reason:

3. Find an animal lover. One who takes care of and raises animals.
   A. Reason:

4. Find a person who looks ambitious. One who gets the job done.
   A. Reason:

5. Find one who appreciates classical music.
   A. Reason:

6. Find one who likes modern rock and roll music.
   A. Reason:

7. Find someone who looks daring and would appreciate exciting activities.

    A. Reason:

8. Find an interesting conversationalist. Someone you could listen to.

    A. Reason:

9. Find a gourmet cook or one who would enjoy gourmet cooking.

    A. Reason:

10. Find a sophisticated-looking person. Go for the refined look.

    A. Reason:

11. Who looks intelligent in this group (you cannot list yourself)?

    A. Reason:

Worksheet 2-6

Professional Conduct

For each of the following professional behaviors, list the professional characteristics or traits it represents.

Professional Behavior	Professional Characteristic
Administering a standardized assessment accurately	Example: Service competency Attention to detail
Offering to put your fieldwork educator's clinical notes back into the clients' charts without being asked	
Admitting you did not complete your notes on time, apologizing, and offering to stay late or come in early to complete them	
Arranging self-feeding interventions pre-dawn or after dusk for an occupational therapy client who is fasting during Ramadan	
Switching a client's treatment time so as not to conflict with physical therapy	
Addressing an adult client by using "Mr." or "Mrs." and client's surname	
Not refusing to work with a client who is positive for HIV or tuberculosis	
Writing a thank-you note to your fieldwork educator after your interview	
Arriving to your fieldwork interview 5 minutes early	
Asking a senator to vote for a proposed law that improves access to mental health services	
Cleaning up water that you notice on floor near the hydrocollator	
Preparing and assembling all the information packets in time for a workshop that the occupational therapy department is sponsoring	
Noticing that the paraffin unit temperature is too high	
Closing the computer screen after entering client information	
Not billing Medicare for time the OTA spent documenting or transporting the client	
Nodding and maintaining eye contact when a client is answering questions	
Participating in an event to raise awareness of a specific disease	
Being the "go to" person for solving problems regarding manual wheelchairs	
Not dating a cute client your age who asks you out on a date	
Ensuring that all the OTA's notes are co-signed when required by law or facility policy	

Morreale, M. J. (2015). *Developing clinical competence: A workbook for the OTA*. Thorofare, NJ: SLACK Incorporated.

Worksheet 2-6 (continued)
Professional Conduct

Professional Behavior	Professional Characteristic
Knocking on a closed door before entering the client's room or an examination room	
Discussing a client's discharge plan with the physical therapist (PT) and social worker	
Acknowledging that the client feels disappointed when the client's son did not come for a visit	
Not complaining when you have to stay late to order a client's durable medical equipment before the client is discharged home today	
Writing several drafts of a SOAP note to ensure an accurate, professional presentation before showing it to your fieldwork educator	
Reporting suspected child or elder abuse to appropriate personnel/agencies to prevent further harm to the individual	
Arranging for an interpreter when the client speaks a different language than you	

Worksheet 2-7

Ethics Sanctions

Occupational therapy practitioners who demonstrate unethical behavior may face disciplinary action at work and, possibly, legal consequences depending on the nature and severity of the behavior. In addition, unethical behavior may result in sanctions issued by state licensure boards, National Board for Certification in Occupational Therapy ([NBCOT] 2009, 2011), and/or American Occupational Therapy Association ([AOTA] 2010a, 2010b). Define the following disciplinary action terms and put them in order from less severe to more severe.

1. Probation

2. Reprimand

3. Revocation

4. Suspension

5. Censure

1. _____

2. _____

3. _____

4. _____

5. _____

Morreale, M. J. (2015). *Developing clinical competence: A workbook for the OTA*. Thorofare, NJ: SLACK Incorporated.

Worksheet 2-8

Ethical Behavior

Determine if the following statements are true or false.

1. T ____ F ____   If an OTA is found guilty of committing a severe unethical act, AOTA can take away the OTA's license to practice.

2. T ____ F ____   An occupational therapy volunteer can report an OTA's unethical behavior to NBCOT.

3. T ____ F ____   An OTA student should begin following the Code of Ethics when Level II fieldwork commences.

4. T ____ F ____   An OTA who commits an unethical act could have his or her name listed publicly as an ethics violator by AOTA or NBCOT.

5. T ____ F ____   AOTA guidelines take precedence over state laws.

6. T ____ F ____   Committing a felony may limit a person's ability to practice occupational therapy.

7. T ____ F ____   If an occupational therapy practitioner did not know about a particular law, the OT or OTA cannot be sanctioned for an unethical act that violates that law.

8. T ____ F ____   An OTA state license is only affected by occupational therapy ethical infractions and not other legal violations of which an OTA might be guilty.

9. T ____ F ____   An occupational therapy practitioner has an obligation to report a colleague's unethical behavior only if it is occupational therapy related.

10. T ____ F ____   NBCOT implements sanctions within 1 week when a very serious complaint is lodged against an OT or OTA.

11. T ____ F ____   A state can suspend an occupational therapy aide's license for unethical behavior in an occupational therapy clinic.

12. T ____ F ____   A person visiting a hospital patient can file a complaint with an occupational therapy state licensure board.

13. T ____ F ____   An OTA accused of practicing under the influence of drugs automatically loses NBCOT certification if reported to NBCOT.

14. T ____ F ____   An OTA receiving 6 months of probation from an occupational therapy state licensing board cannot practice for the entire 6 months.

15. T ____ F ____   An OTA sanctioned by NBCOT cannot appeal the decision.

16. T ____ F ____   Minimizing a client's progress when documenting is not considered unethical if it helps the person receive essential therapy services from the insurance company.

17. T ____ F ____   An occupational therapy practitioner cannot be disciplined by AOTA, NBCOT, and an occupational therapy state licensure board all at the same time.

Morreale, M. J. (2015). *Developing clinical competence: A workbook for the OTA.* Thorofare, NJ: SLACK Incorporated.

Worksheet 2-8 (continued)

Ethical Behavior

18. T ___   F ___   It is acceptable for an OTA to refuse to treat a person with HIV if the OTA is concerned about catching the disease.

19. T ___   F ___   An OTA censured by an occupational therapy state licensure board cannot practice during the time of the censure.

20. T ___   F ___   When an occupational therapy licensure board's sanction is revocation, the occupational therapy practitioner can only practice with daily, direct supervision.

Learning Activity 2-2: Unprofessional Conduct

List several possible consequences for each of the following negative behaviors of an OTA. Consider how the OTA's actions might create specific safety concerns or problems, affect relationships with a client or colleagues, or merit disciplinary action by not complying with facility policy and procedures or professional standards such as the AOTA's *Code of Ethics* (2010b). Under the specific behavior, list the type of trait it represents, such as poor safety awareness, inattention to detail, or the specific unethical behavior.

OTA Negative Behavior	Potential Safety Concerns or Problems	Possible Effect on Relationship With Clients or Colleagues	Possible Disciplinary Action That May Result
Habitually arriving to work late Trait:			
Not putting therapy equipment away when finished using Trait:			
Playing games on your work computer while waiting for your outpatients to arrive Trait:			
Jokingly telling a first-grader that he needs to complete therapy activities now or you will not let that student go home today Trait:			
During Level I fieldwork at a hospital, giving a client your home phone number so the client can call to ask questions or just to talk Trait:			
Realizing that a pair of scissors is missing after an occupational therapy crafts group in a mental health setting Trait:			
Accidentally sending an email containing confidential client information to the wrong email address or leaving a printed copy on the copy machine Trait:			

Morreale, M. J. (2015). *Developing clinical competence: A workbook for the OTA.* Thorofare, NJ: SLACK Incorporated.

OTA Negative Behavior	Potential Safety Concerns or Problems	Possible Effect on Relationship With Clients or Colleagues	Possible Disciplinary Action That May Result
Telling a client that he or she looks "hot and sexy" in an outfit Trait:			
Talking to a colleague about a client while buying candy in the hospital gift shop Trait:			
Calling in sick in order to go to a concert with a friend Trait:			
Forgetting to fill out the purchase requisition for reachers, sock aids, and long-handled shoehorns Trait:			
Not washing hands after treating a client Trait:			
Signing a note written by another OTA because the other OTA forgot to sign it before going home Trait:			
Casually conversing with colleagues while a client is performing exercises or an ADL activity Trait:			
Not informing nursing staff that the client experienced an episode of incontinence in therapy and now has soiled clothing Trait:			
Throwing away draft SOAP notes in the garbage pail without shredding or removing identifying information Trait:			

OTA Negative Behavior	Potential Safety Concerns or Problems	Possible Effect on Relationship With Clients or Colleagues	Possible Disciplinary Action That May Result
Asking an occupational therapy aide to perform a skilled OT intervention with a client because you are too busy to manage all the clients today Trait:			
Losing occupational therapy paperwork that was previously entered in the client's chart Trait:			
Minimizing a client's progress in a treatment note so the insurance company will approve additional sessions Trait:			
Forgetting to bring your professional name tag to work Trait:			
Criticizing a colleague's skills in front of clients or staff Trait:			
A fieldwork educator giving a passing grade to an OTA fieldwork student because the student had a strong work ethic, even though the student did not meet fieldwork competencies Trait:			
Forgetting to lock wheelchair brakes during a client transfer Trait:			
Telling a post-surgical client with poor recovery that his surgeon is a "quack" with a reputation for botching surgery Trait:			
Accepting cash gifts from your client in home care Trait:			

Morreale, M. J. (2015). *Developing clinical competence: A workbook for the OTA*. Thorofare, NJ: SLACK Incorporated.

OTA Negative Behavior	Potential Safety Concerns or Problems	Possible Effect on Relationship With Clients or Colleagues	Possible Disciplinary Action That May Result
Giving a glass of water to an unfamiliar nursing home client when he or she asks you for a drink Trait:			
Forgetting to set a timer when placing a hot or cold pack on a client Trait:			

Worksheet 2-9

Written Communication

Critique the following email that an OTA student wrote to her professor. List 10 suggestions to improve this note.

Hey Prof Jones,

I don't think it is fare that u failed me on my research paper. 😠 *I SPEND A LOT OF TIME AND WORKED REALLY HARD ON IT! I wanna meat with u ASAP to discuss. Thx.*

Mary Smith

Suggestions to improve this note:

1.

2.

3.

4.

5.

6.

7.

8.

9.

10.

Morreale, M. J. (2015). *Developing clinical competence: A workbook for the OTA.* Thorofare, NJ: SLACK Incorporated.

Learning Activity 2-3: Professional Communication

Imagine you just had a 1-hour interview with your fieldwork educator, Nick Knack, regarding your upcoming Level II fieldwork experience. You learned you will be working primarily on the spinal cord and traumatic brain injury units. During the interview it was confirmed that you are scheduled to begin fieldwork on the first Monday of next month. Your fieldwork educator requested that on your first day you meet him in the Human Resources office at 8:00 a.m. to fill out required paperwork. In the space below (or using a computer), write a sample email to the fieldwork educator as a follow-up to your recent interview. Switch notes with a partner and critique each other's notes.

Consider the note created for this exercise. Does it thank the fieldwork educator for his time, demonstrate enthusiasm for the upcoming experience, and confirm the meeting place and time? Is the note free from slang and errors in spelling and grammar? Does the note convey a professional image and include a respectful greeting and an appropriate closing?

Worksheet 2-10

Avoiding Documentation Errors

Rewrite the following sentences to make them more professional by correcting errors in spelling, abbreviations, grammar, and fundamentals of documentation.

1. The client was able to preform wheelchair mobility independently to go from his hospital room to the dinning room.

2. The students musical instruments were stored in the band teacher's office.

3. The COPD client stated she becomes OBS when performing heavy activities for more then a few minutes.

4. The Occupational Therapy Assistant instructed the client on therapy puddy exercises.

5. The PT. was seen for 30 minutes bedside to help her eat breakfast.

6. The client's dysphasia contributed to his inspiration pnumonia.

7. The child needed modified assistance to donn his splint.

8. The client stated "he cannot wait to go home."

9. The client used his bad hand to grasp the bed rail when rolling to the left.

10. The TBI worked on ↓ safety and ↑ left neglect to improve IADL performance.

Adapted from Morreale, M. J., & Borcherding, S. (2013). *The OTA's guide to documentation: Writing SOAP notes* (3rd ed.). Thorofare, NJ: SLACK Incorporated.

Worksheet 2-11

Avoiding Documentation Errors—More Practice

Rewrite the following sentences to make them more professional by correcting errors in spelling, abbreviations, grammar, and fundamentals of documentation.

1. The student asked if the OTA could help her write her name?

2. The resident exhibited urinary incontinents and stated "I have a urinary track infection".

3. The client was instructed in arom exercises so that her bad arm does not get stiff.

4. The home health aid was adapt at transfering clients.

5. The client's throat was sore because the speech pathologist made the client speak two long in therapy.

6. The pt.'s torn rotary cuff required surgery and afterward his deltoid was painful when palpitated.

7. The two OTA's treated the OT's to lunch when they got a promotion.

8. The child griped the toy steering wheel with her dominate right hand and used her left hand to press the horn.

9. The clients' tremers made it unsafe for her to use the parrafin machine.

10. The toddler with Autism exhibited a positive babinski sign.

Adapted from Morreale, M. J., & Borcherding, S. (2013). *The OTA's guide to documentation: Writing SOAP notes* (3rd ed.). Thorofare, NJ: SLACK Incorporated.

Worksheet 2-12

Documentation Fundamentals

An OTA wrote the following note after contact with a client. Use AOTA's *Guidelines for Documentation of Occupational Therapy* (2013) or other documentation resources to help determine which fundamental elements are incorrect or missing in the OTA's note below.

Really Good Rehabilitation Center
Restful Springs, Florida

Name: *Rhezzident, R.*   Date of Birth: *4/1/1932*

Dx: *Right mastectomy 2° Breast Cancer*   Physician: *Dr. Seth Oscope*

11:30: Client in bed and refusing therapy this morning due to side eff. from chemotherapy. Client stated she vomited ~~two~~ three times this morning and is tired from not sleeping well last night. Plan: attempt therapy again this aft. and instruct client on right upper extremity AROM exercises.

J.W.

1.

2.

3.

4.

5.

6.

7.

8.

9.

10.

Adapted from Morreale, M. J., & Borcherding, S. (2013). *The OTA's guide to documentation: Writing SOAP notes* (3rd ed.). Thorofare, NJ: SLACK Incorporated.

Worksheet 2-13

Managing a Schedule

Imagine you recently started a new OTA job with work hours from 8:30 a.m. to 4:30 p.m. You are allowed a 30-minute lunch break and may also take two 15-minute breaks (one in the morning and one in the afternoon). Your caseload consists of 10 clients, described on the next page, and you have a mandatory 30-minute staff meeting today at 11:00 a.m. In addition, you must also set aside time to collaborate with your occupational therapy supervisor and complete all of your daily paperwork and departmental tasks. Fill in your schedule below, including the best time frames for treating your clients.

Time	*Client*
8:30 a.m.	
9:00 a.m.	
9:30 a.m.	
10:00 a.m.	
10:30 a.m.	
11:00 a.m.	
11:30 a.m.	
12:00 p.m.	
12:30 p.m.	
1:00 p.m.	
1:30 p.m.	
2:00 p.m.	
2:30 p.m.	
3:00 p.m.	
3:30 p.m.	
4:00 p.m.	
4:30 p.m.	

Worksheet 2-13 (continued)
Managing a Schedule

Client Caseload (approximately 30 minutes each session)

- Mary sustained a stroke and requires instruction in self-feeding. Her schedule includes physical therapy at 9:00 a.m. and speech therapy at 3:00 p.m.

- Tim has colon cancer and requires instruction in energy conservation. He receives chemotherapy at 1:00 p.m.

- Mabel sustained a stroke and requires instruction in grooming. She receives physical therapy daily at 10:30 a.m. and speech therapy at 2:00 p.m.

- Leroy has undergone rotator cuff surgery and requires instruction in post-surgical care of the involved extremity before his discharge at noon.

- Jim has Parkinson's disease and requires instruction in safe transfers. He is scheduled for physical therapy at 3:00 p.m.

- Leila sustained a left femur fracture and now must use a walker. She needs recommendations for durable medical/adaptive equipment prior to her discharge at noon. She is scheduled for physical therapy at 8:30 a.m.

- Natasha has undergone surgery for a right below-knee amputation and needs exercises to increase her upper body strength and endurance. She receives physical therapy daily at 11:00 a.m.

- Ellen sustained multiple trauma from a motor vehicle accident recently. She needs a right resting hand splint today. Physical therapy is scheduled for 2:00 p.m.

- Mario sustained a stroke and needs activities to decrease his left neglect and improve cognition. He is scheduled for an MRI at 3:00 p.m.

- Harvey is recovering from pneumonia and is being discharged tomorrow. He needs a home exercise program to increase activity tolerance. He is scheduled for physical therapy at 12:30 p.m.

Learning Activity 2-4: Gathering and Organizing Therapy Items

As OTAs are often pressed for time in a work day, it is important to perform tasks efficiently. To avoid wasted time, gather and organize therapy materials ahead of time whenever possible, such as when planning to implement a home health or school-based intervention, treat a client bedside, or assess client factors.

Consider the following clients on your caseload. Make a list of all the items you will need to gather and bring with you in order to implement each client intervention. Be sure to consider any paperwork or documentation materials you may also need.

1. *Home health:* Stanley is a 75-year-old male diagnosed with Parkinson's disease. He was recently discharged from an acute care hospital to home, but never had occupational therapy. Stanley exhibits fair plus muscle strength in both upper extremities and fair activity tolerance. He demonstrates decreased dynamic sitting balance and reports dizziness when bending over. The OT evaluated Stanley 2 days ago and, for today's session, has asked you to initiate upper extremity strengthening and to teach Stanley lower body dressing using adaptive equipment.

2. *School setting:* Tamika is an 8-year-old student diagnosed with a developmental delay. She has decreased muscle tone, resulting in poor posture while sitting at her desk. Tamika also demonstrates difficulty holding a pencil properly, maintaining wrist extension, and staying within the lines when writing. The OT has asked you to work with Tamika in the classroom today and provide some adaptations for Tamika's weaknesses.

3. *Acute care hospital:* Brad was involved in a motor vehicle accident and sustained multiple trauma, including bilateral femur fractures, internal injuries, and a wrist sprain. He is presently on bedrest but is conscious and awake. The doctor has ordered an ulnar gutter splint for Brad's wrist. Today the OT has asked you to fabricate Brad's splint bedside as the department does not have a prefabricated splint that can be used. A rolling cart is available to transport items.

4. *Outpatient clinic:* Margaret is 50 years old and has CMC osteoarthritis in her right, nondominant thumb. Today the OT has asked you to assess Margaret's affected hand for thumb active range of motion (AROM), grip and pinch strength, and to work on fine-motor skills.

Answers to Worksheets

Worksheet 2-1: Scheduling Fieldwork

1. C. Attempts to schedule fieldwork should be made as soon as possible, as it may take several weeks just to connect with your fieldwork educator. Also, although you may want to complete fieldwork during a particular time frame, this may not fit with your supervisor's schedule. Your fieldwork educator may be on vacation, or there may be other students scheduled at that time. If you wait until only a short time before your desired time frame and cannot be accommodated, then it may be too late to complete fieldwork by your program deadline. Contacting your fieldwork educator as soon as possible after fieldwork has been assigned should give you enough time to schedule a mutually agreeable time frame.

2. D. Occupational therapy practitioners are very busy at clinical sites and may not be able to return your call immediately. Also, that person may not have received the message or may forget to call you back. You should try and call again. If you cannot contact your fieldwork educator after three or four attempts over several weeks, then you should discuss this with your academic fieldwork coordinator. It would not be appropriate to ask for the rehabilitation director at this time.

3. C. Due to staffing changes, scheduled vacations, and other factors, the facility may assign a different fieldwork educator to you. You should schedule your fieldwork with this new supervisor, but also immediately inform your academic fieldwork coordinator regarding the change.

4. A. A student should not attend fieldwork with an illness that could be contagious to clients or staff or significantly impact job performance. People understand that emergencies and illnesses do occur but do expect that situations be handled appropriately. The professional action to take is for you to immediately notify your fieldwork educator that you will be absent, humbly apologize for the inconvenience your illness causes, and ask politely to reschedule. Realize the site may not agree to reschedule and, if this is the case, do not get upset or argue with the site. You should also notify your academic fieldwork coordinator about your illness and absence and determine whether or not the site is able to reschedule your fieldwork. If you are planning to see a health professional for treatment of your illness, it is helpful to offer your fieldwork educator and academic fieldwork coordinator medical documentation to verify that you have a valid reason to be absent.

5. B. First of all, do not panic! Fieldwork schedules can change due to a variety of reasons so this is not an uncommon situation. It would not be productive to argue with the fieldwork educator. Your first course of action would be to immediately contact your academic fieldwork coordinator. Your academic fieldwork coordinator can discuss your situation with the two sites and help you find a workable solution. Perhaps the second site can be rescheduled or your fieldwork coordinator may be able to substitute a different site for your first or second fieldwork, although you may need to be flexible with time frames.

6. C. This is not an uncommon situation. Thank the person for contacting you, notify your academic fieldwork coordinator of the change, and wait a day or two for the new person to contact you as directed. If you do not hear from the new person in several days, be sure to follow up. It would be inappropriate to speak to the rehabilitation director or ask the person to switch students.

7. A. One week is more than adequate time to wait for a reply, so you should follow up immediately and resend your email. The fieldwork educator may have overlooked the email or deleted it accidentally, so do not be defensive or accusatory. There is no need to contact the rehabilitation director. You should make further attempts to contact the fieldwork educator before asking your academic fieldwork coordinator to intervene.

8. D. Follow your college's policy regarding fieldwork absences for inclement weather, emergencies, or other situations. You should also understand the consequences for unexcused absences. Health facilities count on staff being present to provide essential client care but, of course, realize that it may be unsafe or impossible for some staff to get to work in severe conditions. Certainly, a difference exists between a "possible" inch of snow versus an active blizzard. Another option is to consider other means of getting to fieldwork, such as public transportation or perhaps spending the night at a hotel (or a friend/relative's house) within walking distance of the facility. The weather forecast may change by tomorrow and may not even be an issue. It would be unprofessional to have a parent or guardian call.

9. B. As soon as you realize you are going to be late, the professional action to take is to attempt to notify your fieldwork educator. However, if you are doing the driving, be sure to follow the rules of the road and only text, email, or call when it is safe and legal to do so, such as pulling over into a parking space. Then, once you arrive

late, accept responsibility, apologize profusely, and promise it will not happen again. Do not lie or make excuses. Lateness, particularly on the first day, gives a negative impression. It is prudent to plan properly to allow enough travel time for unexpected situations or traffic.

10. D. Emergencies and other situations happen occasionally, so you might find that your fieldwork schedule changes. You should remain patient, understanding, and flexible. It would be unprofessional to cry, whine, or contact the supervisor. Reschedule the fieldwork and contact your academic fieldwork educator to discuss the situation. It is best to not wait until the last minute to complete fieldwork, to allow for unexpected changes.

Worksheet 2-2: Fieldwork Phone Interview

1. N. Directions to the fieldwork site
   Working occupational therapy practitioners are very busy. It may be perceived as unprofessional to ask for non-clinical information you can easily obtain on your own. It is better to obtain directions by other means such as the Internet or by using a navigation system.

2. Y. Start and end times for the day

3. Y. Where to meet in the facility

4. N. If the facility is in a "bad" area
   This type of question is not professional and might be perceived as discriminatory.

5. Y. Date(s) to complete fieldwork

6. N. Amount of time for lunch
   This type of question may be perceived as unprofessional, as it implies you are more interested in breaks. You might ask, "Can you tell me about a typical day's schedule?" It may be prudent to pack a lunch to bring with you the first day as there may not be enough time to purchase lunch offsite or wait in line in the cafeteria.

7. N. Permission to come in late because you have to drive your kids to school
   You are expected to be at the site during typical working hours. You should try to make other arrangements for your children.

8. Y. If a lab coat is required

9. N. Wearing of sneakers
   Sneakers are not considered professional attire, so it is best not to initiate asking about them. Plan to wear comfortable low-heeled shoes, preferably with rubber soles. If your supervisor happens to indicate that sneakers may be worn, realize the sneakers must be clean (no scuff marks or dirt), low profile, and tasteful (i.e., no blinking lights, sparkles, or bright colors).

10. N. Availability of coffee or tea in the morning
    Your focus should be on the clinical experience. Plan to have your breakfast or beverage before coming to the fieldwork site.

11. N. Permission to use your cell phone so you can monitor your children
    Your entire focus should be on the clinical experience while you are at the site. While a brief call at lunchtime should be acceptable, it is best to make alternate arrangements for your children for the rest of the work day.

12. N. Permission to come in late or leave early to accommodate your bus or train schedule
    You are expected to be at the site during typical working hours, even if it is not the most convenient for you. Plan to take an earlier or later bus/train or make other arrangements, such as taking a taxi or asking a friend or family member to drive you.

13. N. Permission to leave early to pick your children up from school
    You are expected to be at the site during typical working hours. You should try to make other arrangements for your children.

14. N. Permission to leave early due to a dental appointment to get your teeth cleaned
    You are expected to be at the site during typical working hours. It is not appropriate to leave early for a routine appointment that can be rescheduled.

15. Y. Permission to wear a head covering if required by your religion
    Head coverings are normally not allowed, except for those required for religious reasons. It is prudent to discuss any religious accommodations you might need.

16. Y. What paperwork to bring

17. N. If it will be a very hard fieldwork, because a classmate failed fieldwork there last semester
    It is not appropriate to discuss another student's experience, and this could also be perceived as a negative attitude.
18. N. Reimbursement for gas and tolls
    Commuting costs are typically the student's responsibility.
19. N. If the fieldwork will require a lot of homework
    A question phrased that way could be perceived as a negative attitude. It would be better to ask if there will be any assignments that you might start preparing for now.
20. Y. The types of diagnoses you will observe

Worksheet 2-3: Directions to Fieldwork Site

List five ways to obtain directions to your fieldwork site without asking your fieldwork educator.
1. Ask a friend or family member
2. Use a website that provides customized driving directions, such as www.Mapquest.com
3. Use a navigation device/global positioning system
4. Call the facility's main number and ask the operator or follow the telephone prompts for directions, if available
5. Look on the facility's website

Worksheet 2-4: Dependability and Punctuality

Your fieldwork is scheduled to begin next week. List at least 10 things you can do to help ensure that you will get to fieldwork on time on your first day.
1. Obtain clear and correct directions to the fieldwork site ahead of time.
2. Perform at least one "dry run" ahead of time to determine how long it will take to get to your fieldwork site and also ensure you will not get lost your first day. Ideally, your practice run should be during the same time frame that you will need to travel for fieldwork.
3. On your fieldwork day, allow more time than you deem necessary to travel to your site. This will give you an extra "cushion" of time if you have several red lights, experience road construction, or get stuck in extra traffic.
4. Set an alarm clock or timer the prior evening.
5. A day or two ahead of time, make sure you will have enough gas in the car if you are driving.
6. Check the weather report to determine if the weather may impact driving conditions.
7. A day or two ahead of time, make sure you have enough cash for parking, tolls, lunch, etc. so you do not have to go to an ATM right before fieldwork.
8. A day or two ahead of time, confirm any essential plans such as a babysitter, car availability, train or bus schedule, etc.
9. Select and prepare your clothes and accessories the night before fieldwork, making sure they are clean and neatly pressed.
10. Pack your lunch the prior evening.
11. Gather necessary items such as your name tag, car keys, and wallet the prior evening so you are not searching for them in the morning.
12. If a lab coat is required, make sure it fits and is clean and neatly pressed ahead of time.

Worksheet 2-5: Fieldwork Attire

Always check with your facility regarding the required dress code. Although some settings are more formal or casual than others, attire must meet standards for client care and safety. Realize that in many practice settings, such as physical rehabilitation and schools, an OTA might be standing and walking a lot, going up and down flights of stairs, bending, transferring clients, etc. Attire should be comfortable, clean, neat, modest, and allow for safe client care. "Business casual" means clothing that gives a professional appearance but is not overly dressy or formal. Here are some typical guidelines based on the inpatient scenario presented:

1. N. Scrubs
   In this situation, scrubs would not be appropriate as they do not conform to the designated dress code. However, in some settings, scrubs might be the required dress code for rehabilitation staff.

2. N. Sneakers
   Sneakers are not considered business casual attire. However, some settings may allow rehabilitation staff to wear clean, low profile sneakers.

3. Y. Flat, closed-toe shoes with rubber sole
   Professional and safer for client care.

4. N. Dressy flip-flops
   Unacceptable for inpatient client care as they can be a safety hazard during transfers or exposure to bodily fluids. Hosiery and closed-toe shoes are often mandatory.

5. N. Low-heeled leather sandals
   Hosiery and closed-toe shoes are often mandatory for direct care. Exposed feet can be a safety hazard during transfers or exposure to bodily fluids.

6. N. Heavy perfume/cologne/after shave
   Clients may be allergic or sensitive to smell.

7. Y. Stud earrings
   One or two small, tasteful earrings are usually acceptable.

8. N. Eyebrow piercing
   This does not give a professional appearance. It is best to remove visible facial piercings.

9. N. Head covering
   Typically, only head coverings for religious requirements are allowed. Baseball hats, fedoras, bonnets, etc. are not appropriate.

10. N. Visible underwear above pants waistband
    This looks sloppy and is unprofessional.

11. N. Neatly pressed dark jeans
    Jeans are not professional attire, although some settings may allow them.

12. Y. Khaki pants and a polo shirt
    These are standard types of garments that occupational therapy practitioners may wear.

13. N. Plain black sweatpants
    These are not professional attire and are better suited for a gym or leisure activities.

14. N. Sport tee shirt/jersey
    These are not professional attire and are better suited for a gym or leisure activities.

15. Y. Button-down oxford shirt
    Standard type of garment that occupational therapy practitioners may wear.

16. Y. Dress slacks
    Acceptable, as long as they are tasteful and not extremely fancy or garish.

17. N. Cargo pants
    These generally do not give a professional appearance.

18. Y. Polo shirt with collar and small designer logo emblem
    Standard type of garment that occupational therapy practitioners may wear.

19. N. 32-inch plain gold necklace
    While necklaces may not be prohibited, long chains could be an infection control or safety hazard during transfers or bed mobility (such as hitting client in face or getting caught on something), or clients may pull on it, harming the health practitioner.

20. N. Charm bracelet
    While bracelets may not be prohibited, dangling charms could be an infection control or safety hazard when handling clients as they may injure skin or catch on client's clothing.

21. N. Well-groomed, long artificial nails without polish
    Long nails, particularly artificial nails (of any length), can harbor bacteria (Centers for Disease Control and Prevention, 2011). Long nails may also rupture gloves or injure clients.

22. N. Dark grey suit
    This would generally be considered overdressed.
23. Y. Name tag
    An identification badge is usually required in health care settings per facility policy and/or state regulation.
24. N. Solid color leggings
    These are unprofessional as the only lower body covering. They might be acceptable if worn under a dress or skirt.
25. N. Solid color hoodie
    This is not professional attire and is better suited for a gym, school, or leisure activities.

Worksheet 2-6: Professional Conduct

Resources: AOTA, 2010b; Lowenstein & Duncombe, 2002
You may identify additional pertinent traits/characteristics.

Professional Behavior	*Professional Characteristic*
Administering a standardized assessment accurately	Example: Service competency Attention to detail
Offering to put your fieldwork educator's clinical notes back into the clients' charts without being asked	Initiative
Admitting you did not complete your notes on time, apologizing, and offering to stay late or come in early to complete them	Accepts responsibility
Arranging self-feeding interventions pre-dawn or after dusk for an OT client who is fasting during Ramadan	Cultural sensitivity Flexibility
Switching a client's treatment time so as not to conflict with physical therapy	Flexibility Cooperation
Addressing an adult client by using "Mr." or "Mrs." and client's surname	Respect Courtesy
Not refusing to work with a client who is positive for HIV or tuberculosis	Unbiased
Writing a thank-you note to your fieldwork educator after your interview	Courtesy
Arriving to your fieldwork interview 5 minutes early	Punctuality Dependability
Asking a senator to vote for a proposed law that improves access to mental health services	Social justice Advocacy
Cleaning up water that you notice on floor near the hydrocollator	Initiative Safety awareness
Preparing and assembling all the information packets in time for a workshop that the occupational therapy department is sponsoring	Time management Organizational skills Reliability
Noticing that the paraffin unit temperature is too high	Attention to detail Safety awareness
Closing the computer screen after entering client information	Confidentiality
Not billing Medicare for time the OTA spent documenting or transporting the client	Honesty Veracity
Nodding and maintaining eye contact when a client is answering questions	Active listening
Participating in an event to raise awareness of a specific disease	Social justice Altruism

Professional Behavior	Professional Characteristic
Being the "go to" person for solving problems regarding manual wheelchairs	Dependability Service competency
Not dating a cute client your age who asks you out on a date	Professional boundaries
Ensuring that all the OTA's notes are co-signed when required by law or facility policy	Attention to detail Conscientiousness Reliability
Knocking on a closed door before entering the client's room or an examination room	Respect Courtesy
Discussing a client's discharge plan with the PT and social worker	Interprofessional collaboration Teamwork Cooperation
Acknowledging that the client feels disappointed when the client's son did not come for a visit	Empathy
Not complaining when you have to stay late to order a client's durable medical equipment before the client is discharged home today	Good attitude Flexibility
Writing several drafts of a SOAP note to ensure an accurate, professional presentation before showing it to your fieldwork educator	Conscientiousness Attention to detail
Reporting suspected child or elder abuse to appropriate personnel/agencies to prevent further harm to the individual	Beneficence
Arranging for an interpreter when the client speaks a different language than you	Autonomy

Worksheet 2-7: Ethics Sanctions

The order of sanctions from less severe to more severe is as follows (AOTA, 2010a; NBCOT, 2011):

1. Reprimand
2. Censure
3. Probation
4. Suspension
5. Revocation

Worksheet 2-8: Ethical Behavior

Also refer to any federal guidelines affecting OT practice and the state agency that regulates occupational therapy in the state in which you are working (AOTA, 2010a, 2010b; NBCOT, 2009, 2011).

1. F. If an OTA is found guilty of committing a severe unethical act, AOTA can take away the OTA's license to practice.
   AOTA cannot issue state regulatory sanctions, but can report the individual's behavior to the appropriate state regulatory agency and take action regarding AOTA membership.

2. T. An occupational therapy volunteer can report an OTA's unethical behavior to NBCOT.
   Anyone can formally report unethical behavior. However, the volunteer should use judgment to consider the nature of behavior that would warrant a complaint to NBCOT versus simply reporting unprofessional conduct to a supervisor or administrator at that facility.

3. F. An OTA student should begin following the Code of Ethics when Level II fieldwork commences.
   Professional conduct should be exhibited throughout an OTA educational program, including Level I and Level II fieldwork.

4. T. An OTA who commits an unethical act could have his or her name listed publicly as an ethics violator by AOTA or NBCOT.
    This is the disciplinary action of censure.

5. F. AOTA guidelines take precedence over state laws.
    State and federal laws are preeminent.

6. T. Committing a felony may limit a person's ability to practice occupational therapy.
    Refer to the NBCOT website, www.nbcot.org, and the state agency that regulates occupational therapy.

7. F. If an occupational therapy practitioner did not know about a particular law, the OT or OTA cannot be sanctioned for an unethical act that violates that law.
    An occupational therapy practitioner is expected to be knowledgeable about applicable laws affecting occupational therapy practice.

8. F. An OTA state license is only affected by occupational therapy ethical infractions and not other legal violations of which an OTA might be guilty.
    Committing a felony may limit a person's ability to practice occupational therapy. Refer to the NBCOT website, www.nbcot.org, and the state agency that regulates occupational therapy.

9. F. An occupational therapy practitioner has an obligation to report a colleague's unethical behavior only if it is occupational therapy related.
    For example, an OTA may report a PT or nurse's unethical conduct.

10. F. NBCOT implements sanctions within 1 week when a very serious complaint is lodged against an OT or OTA.
    The process of information gathering and appeals require a longer time frame.

11. F. A state can suspend an occupational therapy aide's license for unethical behavior in an occupational therapy clinic.
    Occupational therapy aides are not typically licensed professionals.

12. T. A person visiting a hospital patient can file a complaint with an occupational therapy state licensure board.
    Any member of the public may file a complaint.

13. F. An OTA accused of practicing under the influence of drugs automatically loses NBCOT certification if reported to NBCOT.
    Any complaint must be substantiated, and there is a formal disciplinary process.

14. F. An OTA receiving 6 months of probation from an occupational therapy state licensing board cannot practice for the entire 6 months.
    That is not the definition of probation.

15. F. An OTA sanctioned by NBCOT cannot appeal the decision.
    NBCOT has a formal appeals process.

16. F. Minimizing a client's progress when documenting is not considered unethical if it helps the person receive essential therapy services from the insurance company.
    It is unethical to falsify or "fudge" client information.

17. F. An occupational therapy practitioner cannot be disciplined by AOTA, NBCOT, and an occupational therapy state licensure board all at the same time.
    Each organization has different functions.

18. F. It is acceptable for an OTA to refuse to treat a person with HIV if the OTA is concerned about catching the disease.
    Communicable diseases always pose a concern for health providers whether it is HIV, hepatitis B, tuberculosis, etc. However, it is unethical to discriminate based on a person's diagnosis and clients must always be treated with dignity and respect. As health practitioners may not even know if a person has a communicable disease, the health worker must always incorporate standard precautions as appropriate.

19. F. An OTA censured by an occupational therapy state licensure board cannot practice during the time of the censure.
    A public disapproval statement does not prevent occupational therapy practice.

20. F. When an occupational therapy licensure board's sanction is revocation, the occupational therapy practitioner can only practice with daily, direct supervision.
    The license has been taken away.

Worksheet 2-9: Written Communication

Resource: Braveman, 2011

1. Proofread written communication. This note contains misspelled words (i.e., correct words are *fair* and *meet* rather than *fare* and *meat*) and poor grammar (i.e., correct verb is *spent* rather than *spend*).

2. Do not use slang such as "hey" and "wanna."

3. Do not use unprofessional abbreviations such as "u" or "thx."

4. Use a greeting or salutation such as "Dear."

5. Use the person's full, appropriate title (i.e., Professor Jones, Mrs. Jones). *Ensure you have spelled the person's name correctly.* This author has frequently experienced students spelling the author's surname incorrectly on homework assignments and emails (i.e., Morreal or Morales rather than the proper spelling of Morreale).

6. Do not use all capitals in a sentence, as this denotes shouting.

7. The use of emoticons or emojis does not give a professional appearance.

8. Consider the tone of what is written and how it may be perceived. This note conveys an angry and accusatory tone.

9. It is better to spell out standard abbreviations, such as "as soon as possible."

10. Use a closing such as "Sincerely."

Here is the same note written in a more useful format:

Dear Professor Jones,
I would like to meet with you to discuss my research paper grade. Please let me know a time that would be convenient for you. Thank you.
Sincerely,
Mary Smith

Worksheet 2-10: Avoiding Documentation Errors

Here are some corrections and suggestions for professional documentation (Gateley & Borcherding, 2012; Merriam-Webster, 2001; Morreale & Borcherding, 2013; Sames, 2010).

1. The client was able to <u>preform</u> wheelchair mobility independently to go from his hospital room to the <u>dinning</u> room.
The client was able to perform wheelchair mobility independently to go from his hospital room to the dining room.

2. The <u>students</u> musical instruments were stored in the band teacher's office.
This sentence does not indicate whether only one student had multiple instruments stored (i.e., The student's musical instruments were stored in the band teacher's office) or if multiple students had their instruments stored (i.e., The students' musical instruments were stored in the band teacher's office).

3. The <u>COPD client</u> stated she becomes <u>OBS</u> when performing heavy activities for more <u>then</u> a few minutes.
The client with COPD stated she becomes SOB when performing heavy activities for more than a few minutes.

4. The <u>Occupational Therapy Assistant</u> instructed the client on therapy <u>puddy</u> exercises.
The sentence may vary depending on the intended purpose or audience of the notation:
The occupational therapy assistant instructed the client on therapy putty exercises.
The client was instructed on therapy putty exercises.
The client was instructed on therapy putty exercises by the OTA.

5. The <u>PT. was seen</u> for 30 minutes bedside <u>to help</u> her eat breakfast.
The pt. participated in therapy 30 minutes bedside for skilled feeding instruction during breakfast. ("PT" stands for physical therapist or physical therapy.) "Help" does not denote a skilled intervention.

6. The client's <u>dysphasia</u> contributed to his <u>inspiration pnumonia.</u>
The client's dysphagia contributed to his aspiration pneumonia.

7. The child needed <u>modified assistance</u> to <u>donn</u> his splint.
This sentence needs a standard term for assist level, such as "The child needed moderate assistance to don his splint" or "The child donned his splint with modified independence."

8. The client <u>stated "he cannot wait to go home."</u>
   The client stated he could not wait to go home.
   The client stated that he "cannot wait" to go home.
   The client stated, "I cannot wait to go home."

9. The client used his <u>bad</u> hand to grasp the bed rail when rolling to the left.
   The client used his affected hand to grasp the bed rail when rolling to the left.
   The client used his weak hand to grasp the bed rail when rolling to the left.

10. <u>The TBI</u> worked on ↓ safety and ↑ left neglect to improve IADL performance.
    The client with TBI worked on ↑ safety and ↓ left neglect to improve IADL performance. Use people-first language.

Worksheet 2-11: Avoiding Documentation Errors—More Practice

Here are some corrections and suggestions for professional documentation (Gateley & Borcherding, 2012; Merriam-Webster, 2001; Morreale & Borcherding, 2013; Sames, 2010).

1. The student asked if the OTA could help her write <u>her</u> name<u>?</u>
   The student asked if the OTA could help her write the student's name.

2. The resident exhibited urinary <u>incontinents</u> and <u>stated "I</u> have a urinary <u>track</u> infection<u>".</u>
   The resident exhibited urinary incontinence and stated, "I have a urinary tract infection."

3. The client was instructed in <u>arom</u> exercises so that her <u>bad</u> arm does not get stiff.
   The client was instructed in AROM exercises to prevent stiffness of her affected arm.
   The client was instructed in AROM exercises to prevent stiffness of her weak upper extremity.

4. The home health <u>aid</u> was <u>adapt</u> at <u>transfering</u> clients.
   The home health aide was adept at transferring clients.

5. The client's throat was sore <u>because the speech pathologist made the client speak two long in therapy.</u>
   It is best to write objectively and avoid criticizing or blaming another professional, student, or colleague in a therapy note (Kettenbach 2009; Scott, 2013). Also, "two" should be "too."
   The client reported throat soreness following his speech therapy session.
   The client reported that his sore throat started around 3:00 p.m.

6. The pt.'s torn <u>rotary</u> cuff required surgery and afterward his deltoid was painful when <u>palpitated</u>.
   The pt.'s torn rotator cuff needed surgical repair, after which the client reported pain in deltoid upon palpation.

7. The two <u>OTA's</u> treated the <u>OT's</u> to lunch when <u>they</u> got a promotion.
   In the above sentence it is not clear who got the promotion:
   The two OTAs treated the OTs to lunch when those OTs got a promotion.
   The two OTAs treated the OTs to lunch when those OTAs got a promotion.

8. The child <u>griped</u> the toy steering wheel with her <u>dominate</u> right hand and used her left hand to press the horn.
   The child gripped the toy steering wheel with her dominant right hand and used her left hand to press the horn.

9. The <u>clients'</u> <u>tremers</u> made it unsafe for her to use the <u>parrafin</u> machine.
   The client's tremors made it unsafe for her to use the paraffin machine.

10. The toddler with <u>Autism</u> exhibited a positive <u>babinski</u> sign.
    The toddler with autism exhibited a positive Babinski sign.

Worksheet 2-12: Documentation Fundamentals

Additional resources: Gateley & Borcherding, 2012; Morreale & Borcherding, 2013; Sames, 2010.

1. No case number present
2. Client's full name not delineated
3. Date of client contact not indicated
4. Time does not indicate if it is a.m. or p.m.
5. Department of occupational therapy not indicated
6. Type of note not delineated (contact note)

7. Initials are not acceptable for OTA signature

8. OTA credentials not indicated with signature

9. Note is not co-signed by OT (when required by law or facility policy)

10. Error not corrected properly (not initialed or dated)

11. Blank space exists between end of note and signature

12. Nonstandard abbreviations used (i.e., eff. and aft.)

13. Note does not relate AROM to occupational performance

Worksheet 2-13: Managing a Schedule

Daily schedules will vary based on factors such as actual number of clients, length of treatment sessions, unexpected circumstances, and actual time spent for chart review, supervision, staff communication, client transport, documentation, etc. In the examples below, the two blank time frames mid-morning and mid-afternoon allow for breaks and "catching-up" if needed. While there are a number of different time frames that would work for the caseload presented, here are two suggested schedules:

Time	Sample Schedule A	Sample Schedule B
8:30 a.m.	Organize workday/collaborate with OT supervisor	Organize workday/collaborate with OT supervisor
9:00 a.m.	Mabel	Mabel
9:30 a.m.	Leroy	Leila
10:00 a.m.	Leila	Leroy
10:30 a.m.		Tim
11:00 a.m.	Meeting	Meeting
11:30 a.m.	Tim	
12:00 p.m.	Lunch	Mary
12:30 p.m.	Mary	Lunch
1:00 p.m.	Ellen	Jim
1:30 p.m.	Jim	Mario
2:00 p.m.	Mario	Natasha
2:30 p.m.	Harvey	
3:00 p.m.		Ellen
3:30 p.m.	Natasha	Harvey
4:00 p.m.	Complete paperwork/collaborate with OT supervisor	Complete paperwork/collaborate with OT supervisor
4:30 p.m.	Workday ends	Workday ends

1. Mary sustained a stroke and requires instruction in self-feeding. Her schedule includes physical therapy at 9:00 a.m. and speech therapy at 3:00 p.m.
   It is preferable to do a feeding session at mealtime. Scheduling Mary at lunch time today should be appropriate.

2. Tim has colon cancer and requires instruction in energy conservation. He receives chemotherapy at 1:00 p.m..
   Tim may feel ill following his chemotherapy, so therapy should be implemented prior to that time.

3. Mabel sustained a stroke and requires instruction in grooming. She receives physical therapy daily at 10:30 a.m. and speech therapy at 2:00 p.m.
   A good time would be during normal morning self-care. The suggested schedule allows for Mabel to have a rest period before physical therapy.

4. Leroy has undergone rotator cuff surgery and requires instruction in post-surgical care of the involved extremity before his discharge at noon.
   Leroy must be seen in the morning.

5. Jim has Parkinson's disease and requires instruction in safe transfers. He is scheduled for physical therapy at 3:00 p.m.
   He should be allowed time for a rest period before or after physical therapy; after physical therapy would probably be too late in the day.

6. Leila sustained a left femur fracture and now must use a walker. She needs recommendations for durable medical/adaptive equipment prior to her discharge at noon. She is scheduled for physical therapy at 8:30 a.m.
   Therapy must begin after 9:00 a.m. (after physical therapy session) and by 11:30 a.m. (before noon discharge).

7. Natasha has undergone surgery for a right below-knee amputation and needs exercises to increase her upper body strength and endurance. She receives physical therapy daily at 11:00 a.m.
   Natasha's time frame is flexible but occupational therapy cannot conflict with physical therapy.

8. Ellen sustained multiple trauma from a motor vehicle accident. She needs a right resting hand splint today. Physical therapy is scheduled for 2:00 p.m.
   Ellen's time frame is flexible but cannot conflict with physical therapy.

9. Mario sustained a stroke and needs activities to decrease his left neglect and improve cognition. He is scheduled for an MRI at 3:00 p.m.
   It is prudent to schedule Mario at least 1 hour prior to his MRI to complete his session.

10. Harvey is recovering from pneumonia and is being discharged tomorrow. He needs a home exercise program to increase activity tolerance. He is scheduled for physical therapy at 12:30 p.m.
    Harvey will require a rest period between therapy sessions.

References

American Occupational Therapy Association. (2010a). Enforcement procedures for the occupational therapy code of ethics and ethics standards. *American Journal of Occupational Therapy, 64*(6 Suppl.), S4-S16. doi: 10.5014/ajot.2010.64S4

American Occupational Therapy Association. (2010b). Occupational therapy code of ethics and ethics standards. *American Journal of Occupational Therapy, 64*(6 Suppl.), S17-S26. doi: 10.5014/ajot.2010.64S17

American Occupational Therapy Association. (2013). Guidelines for documentation of occupational therapy. *American Journal of Occupational Therapy, 67*(6 Suppl.), S32-S38. doi: 10.5014/ajot.2013.67S32

Braveman, B. (2011). Communication in the workplace. In K. Jacobs & G. L. McCormack (Eds.), *The occupational therapy manager* (5th ed.) (pp. 195-208). Bethesda, MD: American Occupational Therapy Association.

Centers for Disease Control and Prevention. (2011). *Hand hygiene in health care settings guidelines*. Atlanta, GA: Author. Retrieved from www.cdc.gov/handhygiene/guidelines.html

Gateley, C. A., & Borcherding, S. (2012). *Documentation manual for occupational therapy: Writing SOAP notes* (3rd ed.). Thorofare, NJ: SLACK Incorporated.

Kasar, J., & Clark, E. N. (2000). *Developing professional behaviors*. Thorofare, NJ: SLACK Incorporated.

Kettenbach, G. (2009). *Writing patient/client notes: Ensuring accuracy in documentation* (4th ed.). Philadelphia, PA: F. A. Davis.

Lowenstein, N., & Duncombe, L. (2002). Professional behaviors. In K. Sladyk (Ed.), *The successful occupational therapy fieldwork student* (pp. 23-32). Thorofare, NJ: SLACK Incorporated.

Merriam-Webster's guide to punctuation and style (2nd ed.). (2001). Springfield, MA: Merriam-Webster.

Morreale, M. J., & Borcherding, S. (2013). *The OTA's guide to documentation: Writing SOAP notes* (3rd ed.). Thorofare, NJ: SLACK Incorporated.

National Board for Certification in Occupational Therapy. (2009). *Professional conduct.* Retrieved from http://nbcot.org/index.php?option=com_content&view=article&id=126&Itemid=119

National Board for Certification in Occupational Therapy. (2011). *Procedures for the enforcement of the NBCOT Candidate/Certificant Code of Conduct.* Retrieved from http://nbcot.org/pdf/Enforcement_Procedures.pdf?phpMyAdmin=3710605fd34365e380b9ab41a5078545

Sames, K. M. (2010). *Documenting occupational therapy practice* (2nd ed.). Upper Saddle River, NJ: Pearson Education, Inc.

Scott, R. W. (2013). *Legal, ethical, and practical aspects of patient care documentation: A guide for rehabilitation professionals* (4th ed.). Burlington, MA: Jones & Bartlett Learning.

Chapter 3

Understanding Professional Roles and Responsibilities

Professional roles and responsibilities in occupational therapy include factors such as maintaining professional credentials, ensuring appropriate supervision, demonstrating cultural sensitivity, and performing services competently (American Occupational Therapy Association [AOTA], 2009, 2010a, 2010c, 2010d). Occupational therapy practitioners also have a professional duty to behave ethically, attain on-going professional development, advocate for the profession, and collaborate interprofessionally (AOTA, 2010a, 2010c, 2010d). This chapter presents worksheets and learning activities to help you understand professional roles, responsibilities, and expectations for fieldwork and clinical practice. Worksheet answers are provided at the end of the chapter.

Contents

Morreale, M. J.
Developing Clinical Competence: A Workbook for the OTA (pp. 69-98).
© 2015 SLACK Incorporated.

Worksheet 3-1

Roles and Responsibilities

For each of the tasks below, indicate if it is a skilled role/responsibility of an OT and/or OTA. For this exercise, assume the occupational therapy practitioner is competent in the designated tasks.

	Task	*OT*	*OTA*
1.	Instruct client in a home exercise program		
2.	Develop the occupational therapy intervention plan		
3.	Determine if a client performs a cooking task safely		
4.	Gait training		
5.	Teach positioning techniques to a parent of a child with cerebral palsy		
6.	Upgrade an exercise program		
7.	Determine discharge from occupational therapy		
8.	Respond to a referral to occupational therapy		
9.	Implement occupational therapy interventions		
10.	Teach one-handed shoe-tying		
11.	Complete the occupational therapy initial evaluation report independently		
12.	Administer a standardized assessment		
13.	Interpret initial evaluation results		
14.	Fabricate a splint		
15.	Customize a resident's wheelchair with specialized inserts		
16.	Administer superficial thermal modalities as the sole client intervention during a session		
17.	Document occupational therapy treatment		
18.	Provide intervention to a home care client		
19.	Instruct client in workplace ergonomics		
20.	Provide specialized instruction in self-care		
21.	Help a student put on boots for recess		
22.	Develop goals for an Individualized Education Program (IEP)		
23.	Assess transfer skills		
24.	Provide occupational therapy in a neonatal intensive care unit		
25.	Attain certification in hand therapy		
26.	Attain AOTA board certification in pediatrics		
27.	Attain AOTA specialty certification in low vision		
28.	Make recommendations to a teacher regarding compensatory techniques for a student receiving occupational therapy services		
29.	Delegate aspects of an occupational therapy initial evaluation		
30.	Write short-term goals in a treatment note as a sub-step toward implementing an established intervention plan		
31.	Update a client's intervention plan		
32.	Write a discharge report independently		
33.	Adapt an ADL device to improve a client's self-care performance		

Worksheet 3-1 (continued)

Roles and Responsibilities

	Task	OT	OTA
34.	Assess range of motion using a goniometer		
35.	Teach nursing staff how to apply a client's splint		
36.	Provide a handout on cardiac precautions		
37.	Supervise a rehabilitation aide		
38.	Supervise a volunteer in the occupational therapy department		
39.	Supervise a Level I OTA student		
40.	Supervise a Level II OTA student		
41.	Supervise a Level I OT student		
42.	Supervise a Level II OT student		
43.	Lead an occupational therapy group in a behavioral health setting		
44.	Observe a child color a picture		
45.	Recommend durable medical equipment upon client's discharge home		
46.	Assess a client's orientation to person, place, and time		
47.	Inform nursing staff about a client's report of pain		
48.	Provide an inservice to the rehabilitation staff about an evidence-based practice article		
49.	Assess vital signs		
50.	Attend a team meeting to discuss a client's care and progress		

Morreale, M. J. (2015). *Developing clinical competence: A workbook for the OTA*. Thorofare, NJ: SLACK Incorporated.

Worksheet 3-2

Supervision

1. Steve, an OTA, was recently hired to work at a facility that has two OTs and three other OTAs on staff. Steve feels he needs more supervision from his supervising OT than he has been receiving since starting work 2 weeks ago. What primary action should Steve take?

    A. Ask coworkers how much supervision time they each receive

    B. Discuss concerns with the rehabilitation director

    C. Discuss concerns with his supervising OT

    D. Wait and see if supervision improves over the next several weeks

2. Huma, an OTA student, is performing Level II fieldwork in a school setting. During the first week, her fieldwork educator asked her to perform various standardized formal assessments on clients without direct supervision. As Huma has never administered those particular assessments and did not learn about them in school, she informed her fieldwork educator about her inexperience. The fieldwork educator responded that the caseload is much busier than normal this week, she is confident in Huma's abilities, and that those assessments really need to be completed. The fieldwork educator also apologized for not having the time to watch Huma perform those assessments this week but suggested that Huma take the assessments home to review them ahead of time. What should Huma's primary action be?

    A. Contact her academic fieldwork coordinator

    B. Take the assessments home to review them

    C. Quit fieldwork

    D. Speak to the rehabilitation director

3. The OT has delegated a client intervention to an OTA today. The OTA feels the intervention is contraindicated for this client, is uneasy about implementing it, and discusses her concerns with the OT. The OT tells the OTA not to worry and insists the OTA should still perform the intervention with the client, despite the OTA's continued uneasiness and concerns. What should be the OTA's primary action?

    A. Perform the delegated intervention

    B. Ask another colleague to perform the intervention

    C. Go home

    D. Speak to the OT's supervisor

4. An entry-level OTA was hired recently to work in an inpatient rehabilitation setting. The OTA is a bit overwhelmed and is running behind with today's schedule. The occupational therapy aide, who has worked there for 15 years and is very good with clients, offers to help out. Which of the following tasks is most appropriate for the OTA to delegate to the aide?

    A. Teaching a client with a recent heart attack how to use a sock assist

    B. Reviewing a client's home exercise program for accurate performance

    C. Asking a client to fill out a leisure inventory

    D. Determining if the client requires any durable medical equipment for home

5. An OTA is supervising a volunteer in the outpatient OT department. The volunteer is enrolled in college and studying to be an OTA. As a result, the volunteer is familiar with how to use adaptive equipment. The volunteer is at the site because she wants to learn more about occupational therapy on her own. It is not a fieldwork experience. Which of the following is most appropriate for the OTA to allow the volunteer to do?

    A. Cut out Velcro tabs for splint making

    B. Review charts to learn more about OT documentation

    C. Teach a client how to use a buttonhook

    D. Provide hand-over-hand assistance to help a client with decreased hand strength learn to use a reacher

Morreale, M. J. (2015). *Developing clinical competence: A workbook for the OTA*. Thorofare, NJ: SLACK Incorporated.

Learning Activity 3-1: State Regulation

Each state has its own requirements regarding occupational therapy practice. Information on credentialing and links to individual state regulatory boards can be found on the AOTA website (www.aota.org), National Board for Certification in Occupational Therapy (NBCOT) website (www.nbcot.org), or by using an Internet search engine. Consider the state in which you plan to work as an OTA and answer the following questions.

State in which you plan to work as an OTA: _____

Licensure

How does that state regulate occupational therapy practice for OTAs?
☐ Licensure   ☐ Authorization   ☐ State certification   ☐ Not regulated

What department in that state has jurisdiction over occupational therapy? In New York, for example, occupational therapy is regulated by the New York State Education Department, Office of the Professions. Occupational therapy in the state you wish to work in is regulated by:_____

_____

_____

_____

What is the contact information for OTA regulatory information for the state in which you want to work?

Website address: _____

Phone number: _____

Does that state require passing the NBCOT exam in order to practice as an OTA in that state? ☐ Yes   ☐ No

Does that state offer an option of a temporary license or limited permit allowing OTA practice before the NBCOT exam is taken or passed? ☐ Yes   ☐ No

If applicable, what is the cost to apply for a temporary license or limited permit? _____

If applicable, how long is a temporary license or limited permit good for? _____

What is the cost to apply for licensure? _____

In that state, licensure must be renewed every _____ years.

What continuing education or other requirements are needed in order to maintain licensure in that state?_____

_____

_____

_____

Scope of Practice

Does that state require a prescription in order for an occupational therapy evaluation to be performed?
☐ Yes   ☐ No

Does that state require a prescription in order for an occupational therapy treatment program to be implemented?
☐ Yes   ☐ No

What health professionals can legally write a prescription for occupational therapy in that state (i.e., physician, nurse practitioner, optometrist, etc.)?_____

_____

_____

_____

_____

_____

Morreale, M. J. (2015). *Developing clinical competence: A workbook for the OTA*. Thorofare, NJ: SLACK Incorporated.

Can an OTA perform an evaluation? ☐ Yes   ☐ No
Explain briefly _____

_____

_____

_____

_____

_____

What supervision requirements for an OTA are specified in that state? _____

_____

_____

_____

_____

What types of interventions are specified under the scope of occupational therapy practice in that state? _____

_____

Are OTAs allowed to use superficial thermal modalities in that state (i.e., hot packs, paraffin, etc.)? ☐ Yes   ☐ No
Are OTAs allowed to use advanced physical agent modalities in that state (i.e., ultrasound, electrical stimulation, etc.)? ☐ Yes   ☐ No
What additional training, supervision, continuing education, or other criteria, if any, are required in that state in order for an OTA to use physical agent modalities? _____

_____

_____

_____

Are there other types of occupational therapy interventions in that state requiring additional training, supervision, continuing education, or other criteria (i.e., vision training, feeding, and swallowing, etc.)? _____

_____

_____

_____

_____

_____

Learning Activity 3-2: National Certification

Information regarding national certification can be found at the NBCOT website (www.nbcot.org). Use that site to answer the questions below.

1. How is NBCOT certification different than state regulation?_____

_____

_____

_____

_____

2. How does NBCOT certification help consumers of occupational therapy? _____

_____

_____

_____

_____

3. How many questions are on the certification exam?_____

4. What is the scoring scale for the certification exam? _____ to _____ , and the passing score is _____ .

5. How much time is allotted for the certification exam? _____

6. What is the cost to take the exam? _____

7. What is the physical address of the testing site where you plan to take the certification exam (www.prometric.com)?_____

8. Of the acceptable forms of identification listed on the NBCOT website, which two will you use for entry to the exam?

    1. _____

    _____

    _____

    2. _____

    _____

    _____

9. Can a felony conviction prevent an OTA from initial certification or occupational therapy practice? Explain briefly._____

_____

_____

_____

_____

10. The initial certification period is good for how many years? _____

11. What professional development or continuing education requirements are needed to maintain national certification?_____

_____

_____

_____

_____

Morreale, M. J. (2015). *Developing clinical competence: A workbook for the OTA*. Thorofare, NJ: SLACK Incorporated.

Worksheet 3-3

Cultural Competence

1. Carl, a 45-year-old male, has multiple sclerosis and has been receiving outpatient occupational therapy. Today the OTA, Cindy, is meeting and working with him for the first time. Carl was accompanied by another male whom Carl introduced as his husband. Cindy has deep religious beliefs that completely oppose this lifestyle, causing personal uneasiness. What should the OTA do?

   A. Explain to the client her discomfort with his lifestyle, but that she will try to do her best to help him

   B. Immediately speak to the supervising OT and refuse to treat the client

   C. Educate the client regarding the OTA's religious beliefs and offer to pray for him

   D. Ignore personal feelings and treat client and his partner with respect

2. Ali sustained a myocardial infarction and was admitted to an acute care hospital. Sarah, an OTA, is scheduled to teach him skilled bathing techniques today. When she gets to Ali's room, he tells her it is against his religion to have a female other than his wife help him with bathing. There are no male occupational therapy practitioners on staff. Which of the following is the best course of action for the OTA?

   A. Reassure Ali that she is a trained health professional and tell him not to worry

   B. Work on pertinent client factors necessary for bathing

   C. Ask a male nurse to teach Ali bathing techniques

   D. Document that the client refused occupational therapy today

3. Chava, a 65-year-old homemaker, devoutly follows the Orthodox sect of Judaism. She is in a rehabilitation hospital following an exacerbation of chronic obstructive pulmonary disease (COPD). Her occupational therapy goals include increasing activity tolerance for IADL. The plan is for Chava to prepare her own lunch today in occupational therapy. Which of the following foods are most appropriate for an OTA to offer Chava for today's meal preparation session, assuming there are no dietary medical restrictions?

   A. Cheeseburger

   B. Scrambled eggs and bacon

   C. Turkey and cheese sandwich

   D. Fresh fruit salad with cottage cheese

4. Parita is 78 years old and recently emigrated from India to the United States. Parita sustained a cerebrovascular accident that resulted in left hemiparesis. She is presently in a rehabilitation hospital where the clients are expected to wear regular clothes during the day. The occupational therapy intervention plan includes goals for independent transfers and safe functional ambulation for home management tasks. Parita is able to use a hemi-walker with minimal assistance, but the OTA notes the hemi-walker keeps getting caught in Parita's sari, her traditional clothing. The OTA discusses this safety hazard with her and suggests alternate garments, but Parita refuses to wear clothing other than her traditional saris. Besides talking to the PT, which of the following is the OTA's best course of action?

   A. Document that Parita has poor safety awareness

   B. Document that Parita needs to use a narrow-based quad cane

   C. Document the safety hazard and client education provided

   D. Recommend discharge from occupational therapy

Worksheet 3-3 (continued)

Cultural Competence

5. Martin is a 60-year-old male who recently had surgery for a rotator cuff repair. As part of the post-surgical protocol, the OTA is instructing Martin on a home program of range of motion exercises, which the physician wants Martin to perform several times daily. Martin informs the OTA he does not think he can perform the exercises during much of the weekend as Martin's faith requires rest on the Sabbath. Which of the following is the best course of action for the OTA?

    A. Educate Martin regarding the medical necessity of the exercises and insist that Martin perform his exercises over the weekend

    B. Educate Martin regarding the medical necessity of the exercises and suggest Martin discuss this with his religious leader

    C. Tell Martin he does not have to perform the exercises over the weekend

    D. Document that Martin is noncompliant

6. Howard, a 38-year-old devout follower of the Orthodox sect of Judaism, is receiving outpatient occupational therapy following a flexor tendon repair to his dominant right hand. Which of the following goals would most likely be inappropriate for Howard?

    A. Ability to hold a prayer book

    B. Ability to don a prayer shawl

    C. Ability to manipulate rosary beads during prayer ritual

    D. Ability to use tefillin during prayer ritual

7. Olivia is a 25-year-old Christian female who follows a vegan lifestyle. She was admitted to an inpatient behavioral health unit with a diagnosis of depression. The occupational therapy intervention plan includes having Olivia complete a project in crafts group to improve her self-esteem. Which of the following would be most appropriate to have Olivia choose from?

    A. A basket weaving project using bamboo reeds

    B. Egg decorating for upcoming Easter holiday

    C. A dream catcher project using branches and wool yarn

    D. A coin purse leather lacing project

8. Eva is a 65-year-old female of Haitian descent. She has been receiving outpatient occupational therapy for several weeks to address her severe chronic shoulder pain. Today when Eva arrives, she informs the OTA that her pain has recently subsided due to a healing service she attended in her community 2 days ago. What should the OTA's primary response be?

    A. Express happiness that the client's pain is better

    B. Ignore what the client said. Based on the client's condition, this sudden recovery defies logic and the OTA does not want to offend the client by telling her that

    C. Tell the client that this seems very unlikely and her improvement is really from the therapy she received

    D. Inform the OT that the client should have a psychological evaluation

Worksheet 3-3 (continued)

Cultural Competence

9. Claire, a 56-year-old devout Catholic, is in a rehabilitation hospital following surgery for removal of a brain tumor. The plan is for Claire to prepare her own lunch today so the OTA can evaluate Claire's safety. Today happens to be Good Friday. Which of the following is most appropriate for the OTA to offer Claire as a food choice for today's meal preparation session, assuming there are no dietary medical restrictions?

    A. Turkey sandwich

    B. Grilled cheese sandwich

    C. Canned chicken noodle soup

    D. Microwavable pepperoni pizza

10. Lin is a 30-year-old Asian male who emigrated to America 8 months ago. Following back surgery, he unknowingly became addicted to prescription painkillers when following the recommended dosage and was recently admitted to an inpatient chemical dependency program. Lin tends to be very quiet during group and does not make eye contact with the OTA. He barely interacts with the other clients and does not openly express his feelings. What should the OTA document?

    A. That the client is depressed

    B. That the client's interpersonal behaviors may be influenced by his culture

    C. That the client is noncompliant with group process

    D. That the client has a poor prognosis

Learning Activity 3-3: Improving Cultural Awareness

Interview someone who has different religious beliefs than you or has a different cultural or ethnic affiliation. Choose one or more of the categories in the table below and compare and contrast them for the two of you. Some suggested topics are presented below. Can you think of other questions you might ask to further improve cultural awareness? Each person should volunteer information based on his or her personal level of comfort for disclosure.

Category	Topics You Might Explore	My Religion, Culture, or Ethnicity Is: _____	Other Person's Religion, Culture, or Ethnicity Is: _____
Appearance and attire	Are there specific requirements or special types of clothing? What types of religious garments/accessories are worn (i.e., shawl, fringes, cross, turban)? Is modesty important? Are head coverings important? What are the attitudes toward body size, tattoos, piercings, make-up, hair styles? Are there gender differences?		
More-valued/less-valued professions	What professions are revered in that culture (i.e., rabbi, doctor, teacher, master craftsman)? What professions are considered least desirable?		
Dating rituals/courtship	How do people typically meet (i.e., arranged marriage, matchmaker, bars or clubs)? What is the length of a courtship/engagement? What is the level of physical contact allowed? Is family approval needed?		
Marriage rituals	Is the ceremony inside a house of worship? What is the type of ceremony? What is the attire/adornment worn by bride/groom (i.e., color of dress, henna designs, headwear, tuxedo)? Besides the couple, who else is involved in the ceremony? What type of celebration follows the ceremony?		

Morreale, M. J. (2015). *Developing clinical competence: A workbook for the OTA.* Thorofare, NJ: SLACK Incorporated.

Category	Topics You Might Explore	My Religion, Culture, or Ethnicity Is: _____	Other Person's Religion, Culture, or Ethnicity Is: _____
Rites of passage	Is there a special ceremony/celebration for transition to adulthood (i.e., Bar Mitzvah, Quinceanera, debutante ball)?		
Death rituals	Is there a specific time frame for burial?		
	What type of services (i.e., wake, Shiva, church service)?		
	Is there a special gathering following the burial or wake?		
	What is the disposition of the body (mausoleum, burial, scattering of ashes)?		
	What type of clothing is worn by deceased?		
	What type of clothing is worn by persons mourning/paying respect?		
	What type of burial container is used (i.e., pine box, ornate casket, urn)?		
	Is there belief in an afterlife?		
	Is there on-going visiting of the deceased's final resting place by survivors?		
Family roles	Who provides care for elderly relatives?		
	Are parents expected to live with married children?		
	Are there gender/family member roles and responsibilities (i.e., matriarch, patriarch, do the women work outside of home, do fathers change diapers?)		
	What are the styles of parenting (i.e., authoritarian, permissive, co-parenting)?		
Lifestyle and behaviors	What are the attitudes toward smoking, alcoholic beverages, and caffeine?		
	Are there dancing restrictions?		
	What are the attitudes toward TV, the Internet, movies, newspapers?		

Morreale, M. J. (2015). *Developing clinical competence: A workbook for the OTA*. Thorofare, NJ: SLACK Incorporated.

Category	Topics You Might Explore	My Religion, Culture, or Ethnicity Is: _____	Other Person's Religion, Culture, or Ethnicity Is: _____
Lifestyles, health, and sickness	What are the attitudes toward sickness or disability (i.e., punishment from God, stoic nature)? Is there belief in natural, holistic, or alternative treatments? Is there belief in cures from spiritual or healing rituals?		
Foods	Are there special foods for meals, holidays, and celebrations? Are there dietary considerations (i.e., Kosher diet, specific meat products prohibited)? Are there religious rituals or special methods involving food?		
Religious beliefs and rituals	Is there belief in a higher power or deity? Are there specific rituals within a house of worship (i.e., kneeling, receiving Holy Communion)? Are there specific rituals outside of a house of worship (i.e., observing the Sabbath, lighting candles, saying the Rosary)? Is there a sense of community? What are the types of sacraments?		
Special holidays	What cultural, secular, or religious holidays are celebrated? Why and how are each of those holidays celebrated?		

Morreale, M. J. (2015). *Developing clinical competence: A workbook for the OTA.* Thorofare, NJ: SLACK Incorporated.

Worksheet 3-4

Attaining Service Competency

1. At her new job, an entry-level OTA is expected to perform transfer training with a particular client who requires maximum assistance. The OTA is unsure that she knows how to do this safely by herself. Which primary course of action should the OTA take?

    A. Ask the PT or nursing staff to transfer the client

    B. Ask the OTA's supervisor for help

    C. Obtain more information on transfer techniques from textbooks and the Internet

    D. Perform a different intervention

2. Today an OTA was delegated an outpatient client who had hand surgery 4 weeks ago. The surgical site is healed and there are no surgical precautions at this time. The doctor's orders and OT's intervention plan indicate that the client needs to work on increasing grip strength and fine-motor skills in order to better manage ADL and return to work. The OTA did not learn about that particular surgical procedure in school. Which of the following is the best course of action for the OTA before the client arrives several hours from now?

    A. Ask another occupational therapy practitioner to treat the client

    B. Tell the OT it is unethical for the OTA to treat this client

    C. Review client's chart and use resources to obtain more information regarding the client's diagnosis

    D. Reschedule the client for another day when the OT's supervisor can be in the room at the same time to supervise

3. An OTA student is performing Level II fieldwork in an outpatient setting. The OT informs the student that students at that site are expected to fabricate splints for clients. The student has not made a splint since taking her skills class in school 6 months ago. One of the OTA's clients coming to therapy tomorrow needs a wrist extension splint. Which of the following is the best course of action for the student?

    A. Make the splint on the client with the OT supervising

    B. Review a splinting textbook and videos

    C. Ask the OT to fabricate the client's splint, as OTAs are not allowed to fabricate splints

    D. Ask permission to make a splint on an occupational therapy practitioner today

4. An OTA would like to learn more about sensory integration interventions for children with autism. Which of the following is the best method that the OTA should implement?

    A. Read evidence-based professional literature

    B. Attend professional seminars

    C. Ask a more experienced occupational therapy practitioner to mentor the OTA

    D. All of the above

Worksheet 3-4 (continued)

Attaining Service Competency

5. An entry-level OTA just started a job at a school setting. When would it be most appropriate for the OTA to stop participating in professional development activities?

    A. When the OTA is fully competent in the current job

    B. When the OTA is no longer working as an OTA

    C. When the OTA has 10 years of clinical experience

    D. When the OTA has 5 years of clinical experience

6. After attending 25 hours of occupational therapy seminars during a current NBCOT recertification cycle, a hospital-based OTA is on a tight budget and cannot afford any more professional seminars this year. To help accrue the remaining professional development hours needed for NBCOT recertification, the OTA can do all of the following except:

    A. Develop a client satisfaction survey for the hospital's occupational therapy department

    B. Supervise Level I fieldwork students

    C. Publish an article in a local newsletter regarding the hospital's occupational therapy low-vision program

    D. Publish an article in an occupational therapy magazine that is not peer-reviewed

Learning Activity 3-4: Developing Occupational Therapy Skills

During your fieldwork experience you are expected to teach a group of clients with COPD energy conservation techniques for home management. Your supervisor tells you that an essential component of the client instruction is teaching them how to incorporate proper breathing techniques as the IADL are performed. You have never worked with anyone with COPD and are not sure how to implement the task properly. The group is scheduled 2 days from now. Consider how you will approach this dilemma and the possible outcomes.

Action Plan	*Potential Outcomes*
Options to address problem	Possible results if options implemented
1.	1.
2.	2.
3.	3.
4.	4.
Relevant learning resources	Contact information for each resource (i.e., library access, specific website addresses, titles of written materials, phone numbers)
1.	1.
2.	2.
3.	3.
4.	4.
5.	5.
6.	6.

Adapted from Schultz-Krohn, W., & Pendleton, H. M. (2002). Learning objectives for the fieldwork experience. In K. Sladyk (Ed.), *The successful occupational therapy fieldwork student* (pp. 11-20). Thorofare, NJ: SLACK Incorporated.

Learning Activity 3-5: Administering a Standardized Test

Imagine you are completing your Level II fieldwork and are expected to administer a particular standardized test in order to meet objectives for fieldwork. You have not learned about this assessment in school and have not yet seen it used in fieldwork. You would like to implement the standardized test properly so that you will pass fieldwork. Consider how you might approach this dilemma.

For this exercise, choose a standardized assessment with which you are not familiar. You might ask one of your academic instructors or your fieldwork educator for access to a standardized test (that is appropriate for an OTA to administer in collaboration with the OT), such as one that assesses particular development in children, visual-motor skills, or coordination. Consider the following:

Name of assessment: _____

1. What steps can you take to become more knowledgeable about this test?

   a. _____

   _____

   b. _____

   _____

   c. _____

   _____

   d. _____

   _____

   e. _____

   _____

2. What kinds of information does this test provide?

   _____

   _____

   _____

3. Indicate three possible conditions that this test might be used for:

   a. _____

   _____

   b. _____

   _____

   c. _____

   _____

4. Indicate the age range appropriate for use with this test: _____

5. Is this test valid and reliable? ☐ Yes   ☐ No

6. Indicate the type of setting where this test may be administered (i.e., quiet room with privacy, rehab gym, playground, classroom, etc.):_____
_____
_____

7. Indicate the general format for the assessment (i.e., interview, gross or fine-motor activities, ADL, visual, constructional, written responses, etc.):_____
_____
_____
_____

8. How much time is needed to administer this test? _____

9. What is the format for providing instructions to the client?
   ☐ Written instructions   ☐ Word-for-word verbal instructions   ☐ Paraphrase verbal instructions   ☐ Other

10. Indicate all the equipment or supplies you will need to gather in order to administer this test (i.e., table, paper, pencil, timer, blocks, leather lacing project, occlusion board, etc.):_____
_____
_____
_____

11. What possible factors may interfere with test administration?
_____
_____
_____

12. Find three evidence-based articles that support or discourage the use of this assessment and cite them below:
    1._____
    2._____
    3._____

13. Indicate how the results of this assessment may relate to a client's occupational performance: _____
_____
_____
_____

Worksheet 3-5

Advocacy

Indicate if the following statements are true or false.

1. T ____   F ____   It is redundant to join a state occupational therapy association if you are already a member of AOTA.

2. T ____   F ____   Occupational therapy practitioners should advocate to help occupational therapy consumers receive the services they need.

3. T ____   F ____   An OTA or OTA student should join AOTA primarily to receive the journals.

4. T ____   F ____   An OTA cannot really do anything about changing a law that impacts occupational therapy.

5. T ____   F ____   OTA students are not able to meet with legislative staff regarding health care reform because students are not yet licensed professionals.

6. T ____   F ____   An OTA can demonstrate advocacy by joining AOTA.

7. T ____   F ____   Although advocacy is important to change laws, it does not impact reimbursement of occupational therapy.

8. T ____   F ____   Social media is not an effective method for advocacy because it is not a professional format.

9. T ____   F ____   Donating money is the most effective way to advocate.

10. T ____   F ____   One method to advocate for occupational therapy is by signing a petition.

11. T ____   F ____   It is very difficult for an OTA or OTA student to know what to write in a letter to legislators regarding current issues impacting occupational therapy.

12. T ____   F ____   Advocacy only affects federal issues.

13. T ____   F ____   The AOTA can contribute directly to political candidates.

14. T ____   F ____   Advocacy cannot impact state regulatory issues, such as occupational therapy scope of practice and continuing competency requirements, because state legislators create the laws.

15. T ____   F ____   An issue requiring occupational therapy advocacy is fair and equal access to health care.

Morreale, M. J. (2015). *Developing clinical competence: A workbook for the OTA.* Thorofare, NJ: SLACK Incorporated.

Worksheet 3-6

Teamwork

1. Which of the following jobs is most important in a hospital?

    A. Nurse

    B. Housekeeper/janitor

    C. Occupational therapy practitioner

    D. Health information system manager

2. The desired goal of conflict resolution is primarily which one of the following?

    A. Getting a raise

    B. Meeting goals in a client's intervention plan

    C. Meeting yearly personal goals

    D. A win-win situation for parties involved

3. The three rehabilitation department heads (physical therapy, occupational therapy, and speech therapy) are meeting to create a new mission statement for the rehabilitation department. On an average day, the physical therapy department provides 100 client sessions, the occupational therapy department provides 50, and the speech department provides 20. Which of the department heads should have the most say in what the mission statement should include?

    A. Physical therapy

    B. Occupational therapy

    C. Physical therapy and occupational therapy

    D. Physical therapy, occupational therapy, and speech therapy

4. An OTA and physical therapist assistant (PTA) are treating different clients at the same time in the rehabilitation gym. No other staff is present in the room. The OTA observes a client giving the PTA a hard time. The client is calling the PTA names and is complaining loudly about the care received. As the OTA is finishing up with the OTA's client, what primary course of action should the OTA take?

    A. Ask the PTA if there is anything the OTA can do to help

    B. Get the PTA's supervisor

    C. Do not interfere with the PTA and client interaction

    D. Tell the PTA's client that the negative behavior is not appropriate

5. During their daily supervision meeting, an OTA and OT collaborated about a particular client and determined the client needs supervision for safe functional ambulation at home. The OT asked the OTA to attend a team meeting later that day with that client's PT, nurse, social worker, and physician to discuss the client's discharge plan. During the meeting, the PT disagreed with the OTA that the client is unsafe. What should the OTA do first?

    A. Tell the team that the PT is wrong

    B. Provide examples of the client's unsafe behavior

    C. Defer to the PT because the PT has more expertise regarding ambulation training

    D. Go get the OT

Morreale, M. J. (2015). *Developing clinical competence: A workbook for the OTA.* Thorofare, NJ: SLACK Incorporated.

Learning Activity 3-6: Interprofessional Collaboration

Considering various practice settings, list several ways in which each of the following professional disciplines or support staff may directly impact an occupational therapy practitioner's role, function, or efficiency for safe and effective client care.

1. Social worker
    Example: Orders the durable medical equipment that the OT or OTA recommends for client's home

2. Dietary staff
    Example: Provides food for occupational therapy meal preparation training

3. Biomedical equipment technologist

4. Health records personnel

5. Physical therapist

6. Speech-language pathologist

7. Nursing staff

8. Housekeeper/janitor

9. Direct care worker

10. Teacher

11. Other:

12. Other:

Morreale, M. J. (2015). *Developing clinical competence: A workbook for the OTA*. Thorofare, NJ: SLACK Incorporated.

Worksheet 3-7

Team Members

For each of the practice settings indicated below, list additional health team members who might collaborate to provide direct care/specialized services to clients or family/caregivers.

Early Intervention/School	*Behavioral Health Setting*
1. OT/OTA	1. OT/OTA
2.	2.
3.	3.
4.	4.
5.	5.
6.	6.
7.	7.
8.	8.
9.	9.
10.	10.
Home Care	*Rehabilitation Hospital*
1. OT/OTA	1. OT/OTA
2.	2.
3.	3.
4.	4.
5.	5.
6.	6.
7.	7.
8.	8.
9.	9.
10.	10.

Learning Activity 3-7: Emerging Practice Areas

Use the AOTA website to explore emerging niches in the six primary areas of occupational therapy practice (AOTA, 2013d). When you have completed the boxes below, indicate which of the niches you might consider working in as an area of practice and explain why you chose it.

Practice Area	Choose Two Emerging Niches	Indicate Age Range Served	Type of Setting (ie, school, client's home)	Kinds of Interventions (ie, groups, environmental modifications, consultation)
Children and youth	1. 2.			
Health and wellness	1. 2.			
Mental health	1. 2.			
Productive aging	1. 2.			
Rehabilitation and disability	1. 2.			
Work and industry	1. 2.			

Morreale, M. J. (2015). *Developing clinical competence: A workbook for the OTA.* Thorofare, NJ: SLACK Incorporated.

Answers to Worksheets

Worksheet 3-1: Roles and Responsibilities

An OTA performs occupational therapy services under the supervision of an OT (AOTA, 2009, 2010c). The OTA collaborates with the OT to perform delegated tasks for which the OTA has service competency, are within the scope of ethical OT practice, and adhere to federal, state, and facility guidelines (AOTA, 2009, 2010a, 2010b, 2010d). Most answers below are based on *Guidelines for Supervision, Roles, and Responsibilities During the Delivery of Occupational Therapy Services* (AOTA, 2009); *Scope of Practice* (AOTA, 2010b); and *Standards of Practice for Occupational Therapy* (AOTA, 2010d). Additional pertinent references are noted in the chart as appropriate.

	Task	*OT*	*OTA*
1.	Instruct client in a home exercise program	*	*
2.	Develop the occupational therapy intervention plan	*	
3.	Determine if a client performs a cooking task safely	*	*
4.	Gait training *This is typically the role of physical therapy, although occupational therapy can support function (AOTA, 2013e).*		
5.	Teach positioning techniques to a parent of a child with cerebral palsy	*	*
6.	Upgrade an exercise program	*	*
7.	Determine discharge from occupational therapy	*	
8.	Respond to a referral to occupational therapy	*	
9.	Implement occupational therapy interventions	*	*
10.	Teach one-handed shoe-tying	*	*
11.	Complete the occupational therapy initial evaluation report independently	*	
12.	Administer a standardized assessment	*	*
13.	Interpret initial evaluation results	*	
14.	Fabricate a splint	*	*
15.	Customize a resident's wheelchair with specialized inserts	*	*
16.	Administer superficial thermal modalities as the sole client intervention during a session *A physical agent modality is not considered occupational therapy unless it is followed up by additional therapeutic intervention to improve function (AOTA, 2012b).*		
17.	Document occupational therapy treatment	*	*
18.	Provide intervention to a home care client	*	*
19.	Instruct client in workplace ergonomics	*	*
20.	Provide specialized instruction in self-care	*	*
21.	Help a student put on boots for recess *Anyone can help a child don boots. However, if the occupational therapy practitioner was implementing the occupational therapy intervention plan, such as teaching self-care skills, or working on client factors, such as bilateral integration or balance, then that would be considered skilled occupational therapy (Morreale & Borcherding, 2013).*		
22.	Develop goals for an Individualized Education Program (IEP)	*	
23.	Assess transfer skills	*	*
24.	Provide occupational therapy in a neonatal intensive care unit (AOTA, 2006)	*	
25.	Attain certification in hand therapy (Hand Therapy Certification Commission, 2013)	*	
26.	Attain AOTA board certification in pediatrics (AOTA, 2013a)	*	
27.	Attain AOTA specialty certification in low vision (AOTA, 2013a)	*	*

#	Task		
28.	Make recommendations to a teacher regarding compensatory techniques for a student receiving occupational therapy services	*	*
29.	Delegate aspects of an occupational therapy initial evaluation	*	
30.	Write short-term goals in a treatment note as a sub-step toward implementing an established intervention plan	*	*
31.	Update a client's intervention plan	*	
32.	Write a discharge report independently	*	
33.	Adapt an ADL device to improve a client's self-care performance	*	*
34.	Assess range of motion using a goniometer	*	*
35.	Teach nursing staff how to apply a client's splint	*	*
36.	Provide a handout on cardiac precautions *Anyone can give a client a brochure or handout. This is not considered skilled occupational therapy unless followed up by skilled instruction or practice (Morreale & Borcherding, 2013).*		
37.	Supervise a rehabilitation aide	*	*
38.	Supervise a volunteer in the occupational therapy department	*	*
39.	Supervise a Level I OTA student (Accreditation Council for Occupational Therapy Education [ACOTE], 2012; AOTA, 2007)	*	*
40.	Supervise a Level II OTA student (ACOTE, 2012; AOTA, 2012a)	*	*
41.	Supervise a Level I OT student (ACOTE, 2012; AOTA, 2007)	*	*
42.	Supervise a Level II OT student (ACOTE, 2012; AOTA, 2012a)	*	
43.	Lead an occupational therapy group in a behavioral health setting	*	*
44.	Observe a child color a picture *Simply watching someone do an activity is not skilled occupational therapy. However, if the OT was assessing the child's performance skills, such as balance, coordination, or safety, then that could be considered a skilled service (Morreale & Borcherding, 2013).*		
45.	Recommend durable medical equipment upon client's discharge home	*	*
46.	Assess a client's orientation to person, place, and time	*	*
47.	Inform nursing staff about a client's report of pain	*	*
48.	Provide an inservice to the rehabilitation staff about an evidence-based practice article	*	*
49.	Assess vital signs	*	*
50.	Attend a team meeting to discuss a client's care and progress	*	*

Worksheet 3-2: Supervision

1. C. Steve has mutual responsibility to ensure that he receives appropriate supervision levels (AOTA, 2009). He should go through the proper chain of command and discuss his concerns with his supervising OT first. The OT may not be aware that Steve has those concerns. If Steve and his OT supervisor are not able to come to a satisfactory arrangement, he might then seek help from the rehabilitation director. While Steve could ask his colleagues about their level of supervision, their needs may not be relevant to Steve's and it could also be perceived negatively as complaining or gossiping. Thus, it is best to speak to the OT directly.

2. A. It is not ethical for Huma to perform those assessments as they clearly require supervision based on Huma's student status, lack of knowledge, and inexperience (AOTA, 2009, 2010a). As Huma has already discussed her concerns with the fieldwork educator without a satisfactory resolution, the next step is to ask her academic fieldwork coordinator to intervene. As a student, it would not be appropriate in this instance to go over her supervisor's head and speak to the rehabilitation director before contacting the academic fieldwork coordinator.

3. D. An OTA cannot ethically perform a delegated task that the OTA believes will cause harm to the client (AOTA, 2010a, 2010c). As the OTA was not able to resolve the situation with the OT, the next step is for the OTA to seek help from the OT's supervisor. Walking off the job is not a productive solution.

4. C. It is not ethical for the OTA to delegate a skilled occupational therapy task to an aide. However, an aide can ask a client to fill out a form that the OTA will review with the client later. All the other answers require professional judgment and knowledge and are not appropriate for the aide to perform (AOTA, 2009; Morreale & Borcherding, 2013).

5. A. It is not appropriate for a volunteer to review client charts as this would violate confidentiality. Teaching a client how to use adaptive equipment is skilled intervention that is not appropriate to delegate to a volunteer or aide (AOTA, 2009). It is appropriate for a volunteer to assist with preparing equipment, in this case cutting out pieces of hook and loop fastener that the occupational therapy practitioner can apply to splints.

Worksheet 3-3: Cultural Competence

1. D. As a health professional, an OTA should respect the sociocultural background of the client and not discriminate based on Carl's sexual orientation (AOTA, 2010a, 2010d, 2014; Robins, 2006). An OTA is also expected to educate family/significant others as needed to facilitate the discharge process (AOTA, 2010d). The OTA can have personal religious values or beliefs but must demonstrate cultural sensitivity, set aside personal judgment or bias, and treat the client with dignity and respect. It would be disrespectful, uncomfortable, and embarrassing for the client and his partner to discuss the OTA's personal beliefs or to offer to pray for their redemption. The OTA should also discuss ethical conflicts or concerns with the OT to become more culturally competent.

2. B. It is important to respect the client's cultural and religious beliefs and not insist that the client perform tasks that violate his morals (AOTA, 2010a, 2010d, 2014; Royeen & Crabtree, 2006). If there is no male occupational therapy practitioner on staff that could work on bathing with this client, the OTA should instead work on the relevant skills needed for bathing, such as range of motion, activity tolerance, or balance. While it is not appropriate to ask another discipline to provide skilled occupational therapy, collaboration with other team members is helpful. However, the OT and OTA might also determine if training the client's wife for this task or having the client's wife present in the room would make a difference in allowing an occupational therapy practitioner to work on bathing with this client.

3. D. When implementing meal preparation interventions, it is helpful for an OTA to discuss food choices with the client ahead of time, as the client may have allergies, dislikes, or cultural considerations. Observant followers of the Orthodox sect of Judaism normally follow Kosher guidelines, which prohibit pork products and the consumption of meat and dairy products together at meals. Also realize that special plates, utensils, and food preparation methods may be needed to adhere to Kosher requirements (Goldsmith, 2006).

4. C. It is important to respect Parita's deep-rooted cultural beliefs and consider the traditional clothing that Parita will wear upon discharge from the facility (AOTA, 2010a, 2010d, 2014). However, it is still important to note the safety hazard and document any client education provided along with the need for supervision or assistance. Perhaps the garment can be pinned or modified to minimize the hazard. The OTA (or OT) should discuss the concern with a PT who has the expertise to assess what other mobility devices might be appropriate and safer for Parita to use.

5. B. It is important to respect the client's cultural and religious beliefs and not insist that the client perform tasks that violate his faith (AOTA, 2010a, 2010d, 2014; Royeen & Crabtree, 2006). In this case, the OTA should recommend that the client discuss the medical necessity of the exercises with his religious leader, as there may be special dispensation for activities needed to improve an individual's health.

6. C. Rosary beads are prayer beads associated with Catholicism, not Judaism. A, B, and D are incorporated into Jewish rituals for males, along with other special items such as wearing thread fringes and a yarmulke head covering (Goldsmith, 2006).

7. A. A vegan does not eat or use animal products, so plant-based craft materials are the most appropriate (Merriam-Webster, 2013). B, C, and D would not be good choices for this client as they consist of animal-based products (wool, eggs, and leather). String and cord are also safety concerns.

8. A. A primary goal for clients with severe pain is to decrease pain for improved quality of life and occupational performance. In this case, the client's perception is that she now has markedly decreased pain, which is the desired outcome. The OTA should respect the client's cultural belief regarding a healing service or other cultural remedies (Royeen & Crabtree, 2006). It would not be useful to disagree or argue with this client. Education or appropriate intervention would be needed for any cultural practices that are truly harmful.

9. B. For Catholics, Good Friday is a holy day requiring abstinence from meat and fasting for adults (of certain ages); limited food is allowed and exceptions may be made for a person's health (Richert, 2013).

10. B. As this client's communication style may be cultural, an OTA must be careful not to jump to other conclusions (Asher, 2006). The OTA's observations should be discussed with the OT and other team members. Perhaps alternate communication methods, such as a journal entry or art project, may be more appropriate for this client to express his emotions more easily.

Worksheet 3-4: Attaining Service Competency

1. B. The OTA should seek supervision and help from her OT supervisor to ensure the client's safety (AOTA, 2009). While the OTA could perform a different intervention or ask other disciplines to perform the transfer, competence in transfers is an essential function of this OTA's job. The OTA needs to learn how to perform transfers safely and, thus, needs to discuss this with the OT.

2. C. The OTA should be able to perform the intervention without the OT directly present (if allowed by state and other regulatory agencies) as there are no surgical precautions, the treatment interventions are basic and very clear, and the client outcome appears stable. The OTA should review the client's health documentation in the chart and utilize resources to obtain information about the diagnosis. However, the OTA should contact the OT if the OTA has further significant concerns or questions—rather than proceeding with treatment.

3. D. As splinting is a conventional occupational therapy intervention (AOTA, 2010b), splint fabrication may be delegated to an OTA with service competency if allowed by that state and other regulatory agencies. Because of the student's inexperience and length of time that has passed since her skills class, the primary course of action should be for the student to practice making a splint with an occupational therapy practitioner at that site before attempting to fabricate a splint on a client (under the direct supervision of the fieldwork educator). Of course, the student may also review a textbook and utilize Internet resources.

4. D. Utilizing a variety of resources will be the most useful for learning.

5. B. Health care, including occupational therapy, is always evolving as new evidence emerges, society changes, and new laws are passed. An occupational therapy practitioner has a responsibility for on-going professional development while practicing occupational therapy (AOTA, 2010c).

6. A. NBCOT provides an extensive listing of activities that may be used to meet professional development requirements for recertification (NBCOT, 2011). Answer A is not one of the approved activities (at time of publication of this book).

Worksheet 3-5: Advocacy

The AOTA website (www.aota.org) contains an Advocacy and Policy section that explains the role and functions of the American Occupational Therapy Association Political Action Committee (AOTPAC) and delineates current state and federal issues and proposed legislation affecting occupational therapy. The AOTA Legislative Action Center (part of the Advocacy and Policy section) describes AOTA's advocacy efforts and suggests ways that individuals can get involved (AOTA, 2013b).

1. F. It is redundant to join a state occupational therapy association if you are already a member of AOTA.
   State associations collaborate with AOTA to address that area's state and local issues affecting occupational therapy. Both have unique member benefits, resources, and networking opportunities (AOTA, 2013c).

2. T. Occupational therapy practitioners should advocate to help occupational therapy consumers receive the services they need.
   The principle of social justice is addressed in the Code of Ethics *(AOTA, 2010a).*

3. F. An OTA or OTA student should join AOTA primarily to receive the journals.
   Although the journals are a very useful benefit, membership includes other important benefits such as advocacy, professional and career resources, website, discounts, etc. (AOTA, 2013c).

4. F. An OTA cannot really do anything about changing a law that impacts occupational therapy.
   The AOTA website lists a variety of ways that occupational therapy practitioners can help influence public policy (AOTA, 2013b).

5. F. OTA students are not able to meet with legislative staff regarding health care reform because students are not yet licensed professionals.
   Students can participate in AOTA's Capitol Hill Day or, as constituents, can contact their elected representatives (AOTA, 2013b).

6. T. An OTA can demonstrate advocacy by joining AOTA.
   Membership dollars help support advocacy efforts (AOTA, 2013c).

7. F. Although advocacy is important to change laws, it does not impact reimbursement of occupational therapy.
   Legislation such as the Individuals with Disabilities Education Act and Medicaid and Medicare regulations (i.e., Prospective Payment System, Medicare B therapy cap, etc.) directly impact health care access and/or reimbursement of occupational therapy services. Advocacy can influence public policy and how individual lawmakers vote (AOTA, 2013b).

8. F. Social media is not an effective method for advocacy because it is not a professional format.
   Social media can spread the word regarding issues. Also, online petitions can be useful.

9. F. Donating money is the most effective way to advocate.
   Monetary donations certainly help support advocacy activities. However, other ways to help include volunteering, writing letters, calling elected representatives, meeting with legislative staff, and networking with other professionals and organizations. The AOTA Legislative Action Center, in the Advocacy and Policy section of the AOTA website, delineates current issues and ways that individuals and groups can advocate (AOTA, 2013b).

10. T. One method to advocate for occupational therapy is by signing a petition.
    Petitions let elected officials know what issues are important to constituents.

11. F. It is very difficult for an OTA or OTA student to know what to write in a letter to legislators regarding current issues impacting occupational therapy.
    The AOTA Legislative Action Center has sample letters that OTAs may copy and send to legislators regarding specific current issues affecting occupational therapy (AOTA, 2013b).

12. F. Advocacy only affects federal issues.
    Advocacy can also influence local and state policy issues. State occupational therapy associations collaborate with the AOTA to advocate for issues such as state occupational therapy licensure laws, access to health care, rights of people with disabilities, and reimbursement for covered health services in that state (i.e., Medicaid, Workers' Compensation, Early Intervention, etc.).

13. F. The AOTA can contribute directly to political candidates.
    Funds must be contributed through a political action committee (AOTPAC, 2008).

14. F. Advocacy cannot impact state regulatory issues, such as occupational therapy scope of practice and continuing competency requirements, because state legislators create the laws.
    Advocacy can influence state policy issues and how individual lawmakers vote. State occupational therapy associations collaborate with the AOTA to advocate for issues such as a state's OT licensure regulations, access to health care, rights of people with disabilities, etc. (AOTA, 2013b).

15. T. An issue requiring occupational therapy advocacy is fair and equal access to health care.
    The principle of social justice is addressed in the Code of Ethics *(AOTA, 2010a).*

Worksheet 3-6: Teamwork

1. This is really a trick question, as every job is extremely important in health care. Besides the direct client services that health professionals provide, other employees such as support staff, cleaning staff, food service workers, health information technology personnel, and other disciplines are essential to keeping clients safe, equipment working properly, and the facility running smoothly. Think about what would happen if bathrooms, medical devices, and operating rooms were not cleaned; the electronic documentation system was not working; food was not prepared; or the facility could not send bills to insurance companies for care implemented.

2. D. When several parties do not agree initially on an issue, the best result is a win-win situation in which the parties have negotiated and each party feels satisfied with the final outcome or compromise. OTAs often encounter workplace situations that require peaceful, practical solutions. Some issues that may cause conflict include compensation and benefits, productivity levels, frequency and amount of supervision, a client's care plan, personality conflicts with colleagues or clients, vacation schedules, office space, etc.

3. D. If the mission statement represents the entire rehabilitation department, the three department heads should have equal input.

4. A. The best course of action is to first ask the PTA if the PTA needs any help with anything. The PTA can then decide if the OTA can intervene in some way or if the situation warrants contacting the physical therapy supervisor. The client may have cognitive problems or a history of violence that the PTA knows about, but the OTA

does not. Of course if the OTA felt that the PTA or anyone else was in imminent danger, then the OTA should take action according to the facility's policies and procedures for emergencies or security issues.

5.   B. It is not productive to criticize or embarrass the team member. The OTA should tactfully provide specific examples of the client's unsafe behavior so that the team can understand the client's need for supervision. It is important to do what is in a client's best interest. In this case, if the OTA knows the client is truly unsafe, the OTA has an obligation to speak up.

Worksheet 3-7: Team Members

The team members listed below may not be present in every setting or you might find that other disciplines are also necessary for client care.

Early Intervention/School	*Behavioral Health Setting*
1. OT/OTA 2. PT/PTA 3. Speech therapist 4. Child development specialist 5. School nurse 6. Teacher/special educator 7. Teacher's aide 8. Psychologist 9. Blind mobility specialist 10. Social worker/guidance counselor 11. Adaptive physical education teacher 12. Vocational rehabilitation counselor	1. OT/OTA 2. Psychiatrist 3. Nurse 4. Social worker 5. Recreation therapist 6. Dance therapist 7. Music therapist 8. Art therapist 9. Direct care worker 10. Dietician 11. Pharmacist 12. Rehabilitation counselor
Home Care	*Rehabilitation Hospital*
1. OT/OTA 2. PT/PTA 3. Speech therapist 4. Physician/physician's assistant 5. Nurse 6. Home health aide 7. Social worker 8. Dietician 9. Clergy 10. Respiratory therapist 11. Pharmacist	1. OT/OTA 2. PT/PTA 3. Speech therapist 4. Audiologist 5. Nurse 6. Physician/physician's assistant 7. Certified nursing assistant 8. Social worker 9. Rehabilitation counselor 10. Orthotist/prosthetist 11. Respiratory therapist 12. Recreation therapist 13. Assistive technology specialist 14. Exercise physiologist 15. Dietician 16. Pharmacist 17. Clergy

References

Accreditation Council for Occupational Therapy Education. (2012). 2011 Accreditation Council for Occupational Therapy Education (ACOTE) standards. *American Journal of Occupational Therapy, 66*(6 Suppl.), S6-S74. doi: 10.5014/ajot.2012.66S6

American Occupational Therapy Association. (2006). Specialized knowledge and skills for occupational therapy practice in the neonatal intensive care unit. *American Journal of Occupational Therapy, 60*(6), 659-668. doi: 10.5014/ajot.60.6.659

American Occupational Therapy Association. (2007). *COE Guidelines for an occupational therapy fieldwork experience: Level I.* Retrieved from http://aota.org/Educate/EdRes/Fieldwork/LevelI/38248.aspx?css=print

American Occupational Therapy Association. (2009). Guidelines for supervision, roles, and responsibilities during the delivery of occupational therapy services. *American Journal of Occupational Therapy, 63*(6), 797-803. doi: 5014/ajot.63.6.797

American Occupational Therapy Association. (2010a). Occupational therapy code of ethics and ethics standards (2010). *American Journal of Occupational Therapy, 64*(6 Suppl.), S17-S26. doi: 10.5014/ajot.2010.64S17

American Occupational Therapy Association. (2010b). Scope of practice. *American Journal of Occupational Therapy, 64*(6 Suppl.), S70-S77. doi: 10.5014/ajot.2010.64S70

American Occupational Therapy Association. (2010c). Standards for continuing competence. *American Journal of Occupational Therapy, 64*(6 Suppl.), S103-S105. doi:10.5014/ajot.2010.64S103

American Occupational Therapy Association. (2010d). Standards of practice for occupational therapy. *American Journal of Occupational Therapy, 64*(6 Suppl.), S106-S111. doi: 10.5014/ajot.2010.64S106

American Occupational Therapy Association. (2012a). Fieldwork level II and occupational therapy students: A position paper. *American Journal of Occupational Therapy, 66*(6 Suppl.), S75-S77. doi:10.5014/ajot.2012.66S75

American Occupational Therapy Association. (2012b). Physical agent modalities. *American Journal of Occupational Therapy, 66*(6 Suppl.), S78-S80. doi: 10.5014/ajot.2012.66S78

American Occupational Therapy Association. (2013a). *AOTA certification: Board and specialty certification.* Retrieved from www.aota.org/Practitioners/ProfDev/Certification.aspx?css

American Occupational Therapy Association. (2013b). *Legislative action center.* Retrieved from http://capwiz.com/aota/home/

American Occupational Therapy Association. (2013c). *Member benefits overview.* Retrieved from www.aota.org/AboutAOTA/Membership/Overview.aspx

American Occupational Therapy Association. (2013d). *Practice.* Retrieved from www.aota.org/Practice.aspx

American Occupational Therapy Association. (2013e). *Q & A: Gait assessment for falls risk.* Retrieved from www.aota.org/Practitioners/Resources/Scope-of-Practice-QA/Gait-Assessment.aspx

American Occupational Therapy Association. (2014). Occupational therapy practice framework: Domain and process (3rd ed.). *American Journal of Occupational Therapy, 68*(1 Suppl.), S1-S48. doi: 10.5014/ajot.2014.682006

American Occupational Therapy Association Political Action Committee. (2008). *AOTPAC fact sheet.* Retrieved from www.aota.org/Practitioners/Advocacy/AOTPAC/About/36338.aspx?FT=.pdf

Asher, A. (2006). Asian Americans. In M. Royeen & J. L. Crabtree (Eds.), *Culture in rehabilitation: From competency to proficiency* (pp. 151-180). Upper Saddle River, NJ: Pearson Education, Inc.

Goldsmith, M. C. (2006). Understanding Judaism and Jewish Americans. In M. Royeen & J. L. Crabtree (Eds.), *Culture in rehabilitation: From competency to proficiency* (pp. 203-217). Upper Saddle River, NJ: Pearson Education, Inc.

Hand Therapy Certification Commission. (2013). *Eligibility requirements.* Retrieved from http://htcc.org/certify/test-information/eligibility-requirements

Merriam-Webster. (2013). *Merriam-Webster dictionary.* Retrieved from www.merriam-webster.com/dictionary/vegan

Morreale, M. J., & Borcherding, S. (2013). *The OTA's guide to documentation: Writing SOAP notes* (3rd ed.). Thorofare, NJ: SLACK Incorporated.

National Board for Certification in Occupational Therapy. (2011). *NBCOT professional development units (PDU) activities chart.* Retrieved from www.nbcot.org/pdf/renewal/pdu_chart.pdf

Richert, S. P. (2013). *About.com Catholicism guide: Can Catholics eat meat on Good Friday?* Retrieved from http://catholicism.about.com/od/catholicliving/f/Meat_Good_Fri.htm

Robins, S. (2006). Understanding sexual minorities. In M. Royeen & J. L. Crabtree (Eds.), *Culture in rehabilitation: From competency to proficiency* (pp. 357-376). Upper Saddle River, NJ: Pearson Education, Inc.

Royeen, M., & Crabtree, J. L. (Eds.). (2006). *Culture in rehabilitation: From competency to proficiency.* Upper Saddle River, NJ: Pearson Education, Inc.

Schultz-Krohn, W., & Pendleton, H. M. (2002). Learning objectives for the fieldwork experience. In K. Sladyk (Ed.), *The successful occupational therapy fieldwork student* (pp. 11-20). Thorofare, NJ: SLACK Incorporated.

Chapter **4**

Implementing Preparatory Interventions

Preparatory methods and tasks, such as physical agent modalities (PAMs), splinting, and therapeutic exercises, are used in occupational therapy to develop or remediate specific client factors (such as range of motion [ROM], sensory processing, pain, strength) and conditions (such as edema and open wounds) with the goal of contributing to the client's occupational performance (American Occupational Therapy Association [AOTA], 2014). Although preparatory interventions can be an important part of a client's intervention plan, these methods and tasks should supplement, but never replace, the use of activities and occupations (AOTA, 2014). With specific regard to the use of PAMs, it is important to note that the Accreditation Council for Occupational Therapy Education (2012) specifies entry-level OTA standards only for superficial thermal agents and mechanical devices. During fieldwork or in clinical practice, OTAs may see other types of physical agents being used in the clinic, such as electrotherapeutic agents. State licensure laws delineate the specific PAMs and other types of interventions that may be used by an OT or OTA in that state (AOTA, 2012). The worksheets and learning activities presented in this chapter address a variety of preparatory methods and tasks used in occupational therapy for physical conditions. Answers to worksheet exercises are provided at the end of the chapter.

Contents

Morreale, M. J.
Developing Clinical Competence: A Workbook for the OTA (pp. 99-136).
© 2015 SLACK Incorporated.

Worksheet 4-1

Therapeutic Exercises

1. An occupational therapy client is recovering from a shoulder fracture. To implement the intervention plan, the OTA is performing passive range of motion (PROM) to increase the ROM of the glenohumeral joint. When the client's arm is flexed to 140 degrees, the client states, "I feel a little stretch." What should the OTA do next?

    A. Discontinue PROM to the shoulder for this session

    B. Continue PROM, but only to 130 degrees flexion

    C. Keep joint positioned at 140 degrees flexion for a brief hold time

    D. Notify the referring physician

2. Teaching a client self-ROM is indicated for which of the following conditions?

    A. Flaccid extremity

    B. Frozen shoulder

    C. Extremity with fair minus muscle strength

    D. All of the above

3. An OTA is performing PROM on a shoulder of a client with Parkinson's disease who has been diagnosed with adhesive capsulitis. The client is positioned in supine with the client's shoulder in 90 degrees abduction. As the OTA moves the client's arm into 40 degrees of external rotation, the client reports sharp pain. Which of the following outlines the OTA's best course of action for the next session?

    A. Document that the client has a low pain tolerance

    B. Do not attempt any passive external rotation beyond 40 degrees

    C. Attempt passive external rotation with shoulder adducted

    D. Move client to sitting position and attempt passive external rotation with shoulder positioned in 90 degrees abduction

4. An OTA is responsible for providing instruction to clients for home exercise programs using exercise bands for upper extremity strengthening. Which of the following instructions should the OTA give to each of the clients?

    A. Perform each exercise for two sets of 10 repetitions

    B. Perform exercises four times daily

    C. Inspect exercise bands for holes or tears

    D. Perform exercises only every other day

5. When using Thera-Band exercise bands, which of the following would indicate an upgrade of an exercise program or an increase in required effort?

    A. Use the same color exercise band in a shorter length than previously

    B. Use the same color exercise band in a longer length than previously

    C. Change from a red exercise band to a yellow exercise band

    D. Change from a blue exercise band to a green exercise band

Worksheet 4-1 (continued)

Therapeutic Exercises

6. A client with rheumatoid arthritis exhibits fair minus muscle strength for right shoulder flexion and no joint limitations in the shoulder. Muscle strength of his right elbow, wrist, and hand is within functional limits. Which of the following would be most appropriate to address this client's shoulder weakness?

   A. Constraint-induced movement therapy

   B. Ultrasound and PROM

   C. Bilateral dowel exercises

   D. Using a tabletop exercise skateboard

7. Which of the following activities is an example of a preparatory task to improve a child's finger to palm translation?

   A. Picking up beads from a table and moving them into palm

   B. Stacking 1-inch blocks with index finger and thumb

   C. Flattening clay into a pancake shape

   D. Using a toy hammer

8. A client recovering from a Colle's fracture is using a 1-lb. weight to improve strength for wrist flexion and extension. The muscle contractions used for these exercises are:

   A. Isotonic

   B. Isometric

   C. Isothermal

   D. Isokinetic

9. A client is using an exercise band to improve the strength of the elbow flexors. The types of biceps contractions used to (1) pull the bands up and (2) slowly release them include all of the following except:

   A. Concentric

   B. Eccentric

   C. Isotonic

   D. Isometric

10. An OTA is working in a school setting with a child who has cerebral palsy. One of the goals in the child's Individualized Education Program (IEP) is to improve the child's voluntary grasp and release patterns for classroom tasks. During a tabletop activity of putting large pegs in a pegboard, the OTA should encourage the child to do which of the following?

    A. Maintain wrist flexion when placing pegs in holes

    B. Abduct shoulder to 90 degrees when placing pegs in holes

    C. Supinate forearm 45 degrees when placing pegs in holes

    D. Maintain wrist extension when placing pegs in holes

Worksheet 4-2

Open- and Closed-Kinetic-Chain Exercises

For each italicized component of the activities listed below, indicate if it is an open-kinetic-chain exercise or closed-kinetic-chain exercise by putting an "O" or "C" next to each.

1. _____ *Using exercise bands* to improve shoulder strength

2. _____ *Turning a heavy jump rope* with another child holding the other end

3. _____ *Weight bearing on forearm* while writing with the other hand

4. _____ *Pushing a weighted toy shopping cart* while walking around an obstacle course

5. _____ *Putting cans in upper kitchen cabinets*

6. _____ *Using 1-lb. weights* to improve wrist strength

7. _____ *Carrying a lunch tray* in the cafeteria

8. _____ *Sanding* a wooden board using a sanding block

9. _____ *Posing like a bear* with hands and feet on floor

10. _____ *Using a reacher* to remove clothes from dryer

11. _____ *Prone on elbows* while watching a wind-up toy move

12. _____ *Rolling dough into piecrust shape using a rolling pin*

13. _____ *Dynamic standing* when hanging clothes in closet

14. _____ *Hanging clothes in closet* while standing

15. _____ *Pressing/flattening therapy putty with palm* while standing at table

16. _____ *Dynamic standing* while using a hula hoop

17. _____ *Performing push-ups against the wall* while standing

18. _____ *Moving rings from one side of an exercise arc to the other side*

19. _____ *Applying lotion* to extremities

20. _____ *Arm push-ups* while seated in preparation for transfers

21. _____ *Cone stacking* to improve grip

22. _____ *Waving a ribbon wand* to music

23. _____ *Scrubbing a floor using a hand-held brush*

24. _____ *Painting on an easel* while standing

25. _____ *Sliding board transfer*

Morreale, M. J. (2015). *Developing clinical competence: A workbook for the OTA.* Thorofare, NJ: SLACK Incorporated.

Worksheet 4-3

Preparatory Methods and Tasks

1. An OTA is working with a client to decrease edema and improve ROM of the fingers to enable independent self-care. Which of the following is the least appropriate intervention to address these deficits?

   A. Using a vibrator to improve lymph drainage in the hand

   B. Contrast baths

   C. Retrograde massage

   D. Overhead pumping

2. In occupational therapy, a client recovering from carpal tunnel surgery is putting golf tees in therapy putty. This task was most likely chosen by the OTA to address which of the following?

   A. Eye-hand coordination

   B. Tip pinch strength

   C. Lateral pinch strength

   D. Hypothenar muscle strength

3. An OTA is performing wound care with a client recovering from a finger laceration. In the initial evaluation performed 1 week ago, the OT described the wound as "yellow," and wound size as "9-mm long by 6-mm wide." Which of the following observations made by the OTA would indicate that the wound is improving?

   A. Black color

   B. Red color

   C. 1-cm long by 0.6-cm wide

   D. 8-cm long by 5-cm wide

4. A client is fully dressed and seated in a chair facing the OTA. The OTA is instructing the client in lightly resistive therapy putty exercises to improve hand function. Which of the following is least appropriate for the OTA to instruct the client to do with the therapy putty at this time?

   A. Squeeze therapy putty into a ball

   B. Roll therapy putty into a log shape on client's thigh

   C. Pinch therapy putty with thumb, index, and long fingers

   D. Squeeze therapy putty between fingers

5. A left-handed 10-year-old child with a traumatic brain injury has increased muscle tone in his right upper extremity and fair sitting balance. How should the OTA position the child when working on graphomotor skills?

   A. Sitting at desk, feet unsupported, right upper extremity in pronation on table

   B. Sitting at desk, feet supported, right upper extremity in supination on table

   C. Sitting at desk, feet supported, right upper extremity holding the pencil

   D. Sitting at desk, feet supported, right upper extremity in pronation on table

Worksheet 4-3 (continued)

Preparatory Methods and Tasks

6. An OTA in a rehabilitation hospital is planning a lower body dressing session with a male client who has recently undergone surgery for a below-knee amputation. The OTA arrives at the client's room immediately following the client's shower. The client is dressed in a hospital gown but the long elastic bandage that has been used to shape his residual limb has not been reapplied. What action should the OTA take?

    A. Rewrap stump using a circular method to apply the bandage then work on lower body dressing

    B. Rewrap the stump using a figure-8 method to apply the bandage then work on lower body dressing

    C. Before performing dressing tasks, contact the PT or PTA and ask that person to rewrap the stump now

    D. Work on lower body dressing without reapplying the bandage

7. An OTA Level I fieldwork student sees an OTA across the room methodically stroking a dry, densely bristled soft brush on a child's arms. The student does not know the child's diagnosis but also observes that the child eventually begins a task of removing beanbags hidden in a bucket of balls. The student should conclude that the outcome the OTA is trying to achieve with the brush is most likely which of the following?

    A. Improved wrist extension

    B. Decreased spasticity

    C. Improved sensory processing

    D. Removal of germs for infection control

8. A client with a cerebrovascular accident (CVA) and left hemiparesis is beginning to get some motor return in the affected upper extremity. An OTA using Neurodevelopmental Treatment (NDT) theory is working with the client on left upper extremity weight-bearing activities to improve proximal stability. The client is sitting on a mat with his affected arm extended at side and palm on the mat. Which of the following is not correct for the OTA to do?

    A. Flatten client's hand completely on the mat

    B. Support client's elbow

    C. Have client shift weight gradually toward affected side

    D. Have client's feet resting on floor

9. An OTA is working with a client using an exercise band to improve right shoulder external rotation strength. The OTA tied the exercise band to a doorknob. How should the OTA tell the client to position himself?

    A. Stand with right side of body nearer to doorknob. Use band in right hand and pull across front of body, keeping the weak shoulder adducted.

    B. Stand with right side of body nearer to doorknob. Use band in right hand and pull away from right side of body, keeping the weak shoulder adducted.

    C. Stand with left side of body nearer to doorknob. Use band in right hand and pull across front of body with right hand, keeping the weak shoulder adducted.

    D. Stand with left side of body nearer to doorknob. Use band in right hand and pull away from right side of body, keeping the weak shoulder adducted.

10. When measuring a client for a standard wheelchair, which of the following is correct?

    A. Seat depth should be 1.5 to 2 inches wider than client's hips

    B. Seat back height should be level with superior angle of scapula

    C. Armrest height should be measured with client's elbow placed in approximately 90 degrees of flexion

    D. The front edge of seat should reach to the back of client's knees

Learning Activity 4-1: Client Factors and Motor Skills

For each of the client factors or performance skills in the table below, list two preparatory tasks and two functional activities or occupations that may be used in occupational therapy to improve deficits in those areas. Examples are provided for each category. Also, determine three additional client factors or performance skills to add to this table. Considering each client factor/performance skill category, determine which of the interventions might be more meaningful or effective for a "real" client and the reasons why.

Client Factor/Performance Skill	*Preparatory Task*	*Activities and Occupations*
Shoulder ROM	Pulleys 1. 2.	Put groceries in upper kitchen cabinet 1. 2.
Upper extremity strength	Exercise bands 1. 2.	Carry a laundry basket containing towels or clothes 1. 2.
Cylindrical grip	Stack cones 1. 2.	Use large-handled utensils for feeding 1. 2.
Hand strength	Squeeze hand gripper 1. 2.	Knead bread dough 1. 2.
Standing balance/tolerance	Stand at table to use shoulder arc 1. 2.	Stand at kitchen counter to make a sandwich 1. 2.
Sitting balance/tolerance	Sit on mat to toss beanbags 1. 2.	Sit on tub bench when bathing 1. 2.
3-point pinch/palmar pinch	Stack small checkers 1. 2.	Put on lipstick 1. 2.
Tip pinch	Put small pegs in pegboard 1. 2.	Put pills in pill organizer (can use beans or small candies to simulate pills) 1. 2.

Morreale, M. J. (2015). *Developing clinical competence: A workbook for the OTA*. Thorofare, NJ: SLACK Incorporated.

Client Factor/Performance Skill	Preparatory Task	Activities and Occupations
Lateral pinch	Pinch therapy putty 1. 2.	Hang towels on a clothesline using clothespins 1. 2.
Dexterity/in-hand manipulation	Pick up foam cubes one at a time and hold in palm 1. 2.	Sort a handful of coins into wrappers 1. 2.
Other:	1. 2.	1. 2.
Other:	1. 2.	1. 2.
Other:	1. 2.	1. 2.

Learning Activity 4-2: Cognitive and Perceptual Skills

For each of the client factors or performance skills in the table below, list two preparatory tasks and two functional activities or occupations that may be used in occupational therapy to improve deficits in those areas. Examples are provided for each category. Also, determine three additional client factors or performance skills to add to this table. Considering each client factor/performance skill category, determine which of the interventions might be more meaningful or effective for a "real" client and the reasons why.

Client Factor/Performance Skill	Preparatory Task	Activities and Occupations
Crossing midline	Moving rings on a shoulder arc from one side to the other 1. 2.	Move kitchen utensils from dish drainer to drawer on opposite side 1. 2.
Spatial relations	Follow a pattern using blocks 1. 2.	Place cookie dough evenly spaced on a cookie sheet 1. 2.
Bilateral integration	Upper extremity pedal exerciser 1. 2.	Buttoning a shirt 1. 2.
Short-term memory	Memory matching game 1. 2.	Use calendar to find/schedule appointments 1. 2.
Categorization	Sort shapes 1. 2.	Sort utensils into a divided utensil tray 1. 2.
Sequencing	Sequencing cards 1. 2.	Follow a recipe 1. 2.
Calculation skills	Math worksheets 1. 2.	Use a restaurant menu and calculate cost of a meal including tax and tip 1. 2.
Problem solving	Logic puzzles 1. 2.	Role-play emergency situations 1. 2.

Client Factor/Performance Skill	Preparatory Task	Activities and Occupations
Body scheme	Orient felt body pieces on a felt board 1. 2.	Dressing 1. 2.
Awareness of left visual field	Pick up beanbags on right side and place in bucket on left side 1. 2.	Locate grooming items on left side of counter when brushing teeth 1. 2.
Other:	1. 2.	1. 2.
Other:	1. 2.	1. 2.
Other:	1. 2.	1. 2.

Worksheet 4-4

Physical Agent Modality Categories

Indicate the pertinent category for each of the physical agent modalities or devices listed below.

	Physical Agent Modality	*Superficial Thermal Agent*	*Deep Thermal Agent*	*Electrotherapeutic Agent*	*Mechanical Device*
1.	Fluidotherapy				
2.	Transcutaneous electrical nerve stimulation (TENS)				
3.	Iontophoresis				
4.	Hot pack				
5.	Ultrasound				
6.	Whirlpool				
7.	Vasopneumatic device				
8.	Cryotherapy				
9.	Neuromuscular electrical stimulation (NMES)				
10.	Functional electrical stimulation (FES)				
11.	Continuous passive motion (CPM)				
12.	Paraffin				
13.	High-voltage pulsed current (HVPC)				
14.	Cold pack				
15.	Hydrotherapy				
16.	Phonophoresis				
17.	Short-wave diathermy				
18.	Vapocoolant spray				
19.	Infrared				
20.	Lymphedema pump				

Worksheet 4-5

Selecting Physical Agent Modalities

For each of the client conditions indicated below, choose an appropriate modality or device from the following list. Only use each modality once.

A. Whirlpool
B. CPM
C. Ultrasound
D. Fluidotherapy
E. Vasopneumatic pump
F. TENS
G. NMES
H. Cold pack
I. Hot pack
J. Paraffin
K. Iontophoresis
L. Biofeedback

1. _____ Acute PIP hyperextension injury with pain and edema

2. _____ Shoulder stiffness due to rheumatoid arthritis

3. _____ Muscle reeducation to learn how to minimize involuntary upper trapezius muscle contraction

4. _____ Healed carpal tunnel release with stiffness, fair light touch sensation, intact protective sensation, and scar hypersensitivity

5. _____ Thumb CMC arthritis with pain and stiffness

6. _____ Manage edema following soft tissue trauma

7. _____ Open wound requiring debridement

8. _____ Chronic biceps pain upon discharge from occupational therapy

9. _____ Conditions requiring mechanical PROM

10. _____ Lateral epicondylitis requiring topical medication delivery through the skin

11. _____ CVA with hemiparesis and shoulder subluxation

12. _____ PIP joint contracture and scar adhesions following a healed laceration to volar index finger

Worksheet 4-6

Using Physical Agent Modalities Safely

1. Which of the following conditions would be most appropriate for paraffin?

   A. Wrist fracture resulting in pitting hand edema after cast removal

   B. Crush injury to hand resulting in digital stiffness and poor protective sensation

   C. Healed flexor tendon repair of index and long fingers resulting in tendon tightness

   D. Laceration of thumb with sutures in place and decreased thumb ROM

2. An outpatient with a shoulder condition requires superficial heat to decrease shoulder stiffness. Before placing a hot pack on the client, the OTA should do which of the following?

   A. Ask client to remove watch and rings

   B. Use an anti-static mat under client to prevent electric shocks

   C. Wrap the hot pack with a terrycloth cover and place a plastic bag over it

   D. Check hydrocollator temperature

3. Which of the following is the primary action an OTA should take when a client tells the OTA that a hot pack feels too hot?

   A. Lower temperature of hydrocollator

   B. Inform the client that the heat will gradually dissipate

   C. Remove hot pack

   D. Find the OT to notify her of the situation

4. Which of the following conditions would be most appropriate for Fluidotherapy?

   A. Rheumatoid arthritis flare-up causing painful hand and swollen joints

   B. Thumb CMC joint stiffness secondary to osteoarthritis

   C. Healed deltoid tendon repair resulting in pain and stiffness but no sensory loss

   D. Shoulder contracture secondary to complex regional pain syndrome

5. When using a cryotherapy gel pack on a client, the OTA should do which of the following?

   A. Place it directly on the affected area without using a cover on gel pack

   B. When done, put the gel pack immediately back in the heating unit so it stays hot for the next client

   C. Cover it with a towel and then put it over an insensate area

   D. Explain that the client may experience a numb sensation

6. An inpatient client is morbidly obese and requires a mechanical lift to transfer him out of bed. He rolls side to side using bed rails, but cannot roll onto his stomach. The client also has pain in his posterior deltoid, for which the doctor ordered occupational therapy, including hot packs. For the past 2 days the client has received hot packs on his shoulder while sitting in a chair. Today, when the OTA arrives with the hot pack, the mechanical lift is not available. What should the OTA do?

   A. Place the hot pack underneath the client's shoulder with client supine

   B. Place the hot pack on the client's shoulder with client side-lying

   C. Place the hot pack on the client's shoulder with client prone

   D. Do not use a hot pack at this time

Worksheet 4-6 (continued)

Using Physical Agent Modalities Safely

7. When administering a paraffin treatment to a client who has stiffness in digits and intact skin, the OTA should do which of the following:

    A. Ask client to perform finger active range of motion (AROM) in paraffin bath

    B. Ask client to wash and dry hands before using paraffin

    C. Place a plastic bag over client's hand then dip in paraffin and cover with a towel

    D. Ask client to immerse hand to the bottom of the unit

8. An occupational therapy client with a wrist sprain has been receiving hot packs to his wrist followed by ROM and functional activities. Today he is being treated by the OTA. When the client arrives, the OTA notices the client has bad sunburn on his upper extremities, including his wrist. What primary action should the OTA take?

    A. Administer a cold pack, then a hot pack followed by ROM and functional activities

    B. Defer treatment for today

    C. Defer hot pack and perform functional activities

    D. Call the client's physician

9. An occupational therapy client recently had surgery to remove basal cell carcinoma from his wrist and is presently receiving radiation to eliminate possible remaining malignant cells. The client presents with decreased ROM and reports wrist pain. Which of the following modalities would be indicated for this client?

    A. Hot pack

    B. Paraffin

    C. Hot pack and ultrasound

    D. None

10. Which of the following situations is most appropriate for cryotherapy?

    A. Client with an acute wrist sprain and history of a carpal tunnel release 6 months ago

    B. Client with Raynaud's and acute thumb tendinitis

    C. Client with upper extremity peripheral vascular disease and acute finger sprain

    D. Client with an elbow contracture secondary to biceps tendon tightness

Morreale, M. J. (2015). *Developing clinical competence: A workbook for the OTA.* Thorofare, NJ: SLACK Incorporated.

Worksheet 4-7

Physical Agent Modality Basics

1. An OTA is working in a state that does not restrict occupational therapy practitioners from using PAMs. The OTA and her OT supervisor are competent in the use of superficial and deep thermal agents and electrotherapeutic modalities. Which of the following intervention plans is not considered occupational therapy?

    A. Hot pack to shoulder, paraffin to hand, contrast baths

    B. PROM, NMES, home management tasks

    C. Hot pack, TENS, home management tasks

    D. Ultrasound, scar massage, BADL

2. Which of the following physical agent modalities transfer heat strictly by conduction?

    A. Fluidotherapy and hot packs

    B. Ultrasound and paraffin

    C. Paraffin and hot packs

    D. Fluidotherapy and ultrasound

3. Which of the following temperature ranges for paraffin are appropriate for use with a client?

    A. 98 to 100 degrees

    B. 134 to 138 degrees

    C. 122 to 124 degrees

    D. 108 to 112 degrees

4. Which of the following is the technique of using ultrasound to deliver medication through the skin?

    A. NMES

    B. TENS

    C. Iontophoresis

    D. Phonophoresis

5. An OTA is working in a state that, regarding PAMs, allows OTAs to only use superficial thermal agents. The client has a diagnosis of carpal tunnel release and the occupational therapy intervention plan includes ultrasound, Fluidotherapy, and TENS. Which of the following should the OTA use with the client to decrease pain and improve ROM?

    A. Fluidotherapy

    B. Fluidotherapy and TENS

    C. Fluidotherapy, ultrasound, and TENS

    D. None of the above

Morreale, M. J. (2015). *Developing clinical competence: A workbook for the OTA*. Thorofare, NJ: SLACK Incorporated.

Worksheet 4-7 (continued)

Physical Agent Modality Basics

6. A client is recovering from a laceration to the hand. Sutures were removed 1 week ago and the wound is healed, but the scar is hypersensitive. The client also has decreased finger ROM and diffuse hand edema. Which of the following PAMs would likely be most useful?

    A. Fluidotherapy

    B. Paraffin

    C. Hot pack

    D. None of the above

7. An OTA who is competent in administering TENS has moved to a new state that prohibits OTAs from using electrotherapeutic agents. The sole OT at her facility is not competent in administering TENS. However, an occupational therapy client diagnosed with complex regional pain syndrome would really benefit from TENS in order to manage severe upper extremity pain. The prescription from the doctor says "PAMs PRN." What should the OTA do?

    A. The OTA should administer TENS only under the supervision of a PT

    B. Ask the doctor to write a prescription specifically for TENS for occupational therapy

    C. Have the OT administer TENS with the OTA supervising

    D. Do not use TENS

8. The OT intervention plan for a client with a PIP dislocation injury includes the following PAMs PRN: hot packs, Fluidotherapy, and cold packs. Today the client informs the OTA that she receives paraffin to her hands when getting manicures at the nail salon and enjoys it very much. The OTA feels that paraffin would be very beneficial to decrease the client's finger stiffness today. What should the OTA do during today's session?

    A. Call the client's physician to obtain a prescription for paraffin

    B. Administer paraffin and notify the OT

    C. Document what the client said and administer paraffin

    D. Administer hot pack or Fluidotherapy

9. A client with thumb tendinitis is at the reconditioning phase in occupational therapy. During a treatment session, which of the following is most likely the proper sequence of interventions for this client?

    A. Hot pack, therapeutic activities, paraffin

    B. Hot pack, therapeutic activities, cold pack

    C. Paraffin, therapeutic activities, hot pack, cold pack

    D. Paraffin, therapeutic activities, hot pack

10. Following a client's paraffin treatment, what should the OTA do with the used wax?

    A. Put it back in the paraffin unit

    B. Give it to the client to use at home for hand exercises

    C. Throw it away

    D. Show it to the OT

Learning Activity 4-3: Generating Treatment Interventions

One of the unique aspects of occupational therapy is the occupational therapy practitioner's ability to use everyday objects for therapeutic purposes. In the spaces below, list specific ways that a **deck of cards** might be used to improve the various client factors or performance skills delineated in the *Occupational Therapy Practice Framework* (AOTA, 2014). Examples are provided for each category.

Joint, Bone, and Muscle Functions

Example: Improve ROM of the elbow—Deal cards across the table to a partner

1. _____
   _____
2. _____
   _____
3. _____
   _____

Motor Skills

Example: Improve standing tolerance—Stand at table to play Solitaire for a designated length of time

1. _____
   _____
2. _____
   _____
3. _____
   _____

Emotional Regulation/Social Interaction Skills

Example: Improve frustration tolerance—Play a card game and wait patiently for one's turn

1. _____
   _____
2. _____
   _____
3. _____
   _____

Mental Functions/Process Skills

Example: Improve counting and math skills—Count a deck of cards accurately

1. _____
   _____
2. _____
   _____
3. _____
   _____

Learning Activity 4-4: Generating More Treatment Interventions

This exercise will require you to think creatively. One of the unique aspects of occupational therapy is the occupational therapy practitioner's ability to use everyday objects for therapeutic purposes. In the box below, list specific ways that **paper clips** might be used to improve the various client factors and performance skills delineated in the *Occupational Therapy Practice Framework* (AOTA, 2014). Examples are provided for each category.

Joint, Bone, and Muscle Functions

Example: Improve tip pinch strength—Use index finger and thumb to push paper clips vertically into therapy putty

1. _____

2. _____

3. _____

Motor Skills

Example: Improve bilateral integration—Stabilize paper on the table while attaching paper clips with the other hand

1. _____

2. _____

3. _____

Social Interaction Skills

Example: Improve interpersonal skills—Ask a worker in office supply store where the paper clips are located

1. _____

2. _____

3. _____

Mental Functions/Process Skills

Example: Safety awareness—Avoid putting paper clips in mouth while working on a craft project

1. _____

2. _____

3. _____

Learning Activity 4-5: Generating Creative Treatment Interventions

The media used in this exercise will require a bit more thinking "outside of the box." As previously noted, one of the unique aspects of occupational therapy is the occupational therapy practitioner's ability to use everyday objects for therapeutic purposes. In the spaces below, list specific ways that a **container of uncooked rice** might be used to improve various client factors, performance skills, and occupations delineated in the *Occupational Therapy Practice Framework* (AOTA, 2014). Examples are provided for each category.

Joint, Bone, and Muscle Functions

Example: Improve upper extremity strength—Carry a 5-lb. bag of rice

1. _____
   _____
2. _____
   _____
3. _____
   _____

Motor Skills

Example: Improve coordination—Move spoonfuls of rice from one container to another without spilling

1. _____
   _____
2. _____
   _____
3. _____
   _____

Sensory Functions

Example: Reduce tactile hypersensitivity—Locate objects embedded in rice

1. _____
   _____
2. _____
   _____
3. _____
   _____

Social Interaction Skills

Example: Express feelings—Discuss significance of rice in one's own culture (i.e., rice and beans, fried rice, rice pudding, etc.)

1. _____
   _____
2. _____
   _____
3. _____
   _____

Mental Functions/Process Skills

Example: Improve measuring skills—Measure specified amounts of rice accurately

1. _____

2. _____

3. _____

Occupations (BADL/IADL)

Example: Improve meal preparation skills—Follow a recipe to make beans and rice for lunch

1. _____

2. _____

3. _____

4. _____

5. _____

6. _____

Occupations (Play)

Example: Improve imaginary play skills—Collaborate with another person and use rice to create a "beach" scene: decorating with shells, hidden "treasure," and dolls "suntanning"

1. _____

2. _____

3. _____

4. _____

5. _____

6. _____

Worksheet 4-8

Selecting Splint Interventions

Match each of the splints or devices below to one of the conditions that follow. Use each term only once.

A. Resting hand splint

B. MP extension blocking splint

C. Airplane splint

D. Palm protector

E. Short opponens splint

F. Dorsal blocking splint

G. Forearm-based thumb spica splint

H. Figure-8 finger splint

I. Dynamic MP extension splint

J. Ulnar deviation splint

K. Volar wrist cock-up splint

L. Anterior elbow splint

M. PIP extension splint

N. Forearm-based dorsal extension splint

O. DIP extension splint

P. Ulnar gutter splint

Q. Counterforce brace

R. Body-powered prosthesis

S. Composite flexion splint

T. Tenodesis splint

1. _____ Carpal tunnel syndrome

2. _____ Boutonniere deformity ring finger

3. _____ Upper extremity amputation

4. _____ Small finger metacarpal fracture

5. _____ Dupuytren's release

6. _____ C6-C7 spinal cord injury

7. _____ Flexor tendon repair of digits

8. _____ Brachial plexus injury

9. _____ Swan neck deformity

10. _____ Mallet finger

11. _____ Low level ulnar nerve injury

12. _____ Burns to hand/wrist

Worksheet 4-8 (continued)

Selecting Splint Interventions

13. _____ Extrinsic extensor tightness of digits

14. _____ De Quervain's tenosynovitis

15. _____ Elbow flexion contracture

16. _____ MP joints requiring realignment secondary to rheumatoid arthritis

17. _____ Flexed digits of a client with end-stage dementia causing skin breakdown in hand

18. _____ Low level median nerve injury

19. _____ Lateral epicondylitis

20. _____ Radial nerve palsy

Worksheet 4-9

Splinting Basics

1. When fabricating a volar wrist extension splint for a client with a wrist sprain, an OTA must mold it carefully to avoid future skin breakdown at which of the following bony prominences:
   A. Radial head
   B. PIP joints
   C. Ulnar styloid
   D. Olecranon

2. A client with an unhealed fracture complains that he is perspiring under his splint. The OTA may take the following actions except:
   A. Punch air holes in the splint
   B. Provide washable cotton liners
   C. Discontinue splint
   D. Instruct client how to clean splint

3. When fabricating a splint, the primary reason for making a paper pattern is:
   A. To avoid wasting expensive thermoplastic material
   B. To help ensure proper splint size and fit
   C. To keep the pattern in the client's chart
   D. To avoid pen or pencil marks on thermoplastic material

4. After softening thermoplastic material in hot water for splint fabrication, what should the OTA do next?
   A. Wait several minutes following removal from hot water then place on client
   B. Immediately place on client upon removal from hot water
   C. Wait 15 seconds upon removal from hot water then place on client
   D. Cool thermoplastic until comfortable and safe for client to tolerate

5. When fabricating a resting hand splint for a client with a flaccid extremity, the thumb should generally be positioned in:
   A. Palmar abduction
   B. Full adduction
   C. Full radial abduction
   D. 70 degrees MP flexion

Worksheet 4-9 (continued)

Splinting Basics

6. When fabricating a splint to address an index finger mallet injury, which of the following is not correct?

    A. Conform splint to transverse and longitudinal arches of palm

    B. Allow for full active MP flexion

    C. Position DIP in extension

    D. Leave thumb free

7. When fabricating a forearm-based thumb spica splint for a client with thumb CMC arthritis, which of the following principles does not apply?

    A. Splint should be half the length of the forearm

    B. Conform to transverse and longitudinal arches

    C. Allow full thumb IP AROM

    D. Do not immobilize MP joints of other digits

8. A client diagnosed with a right CVA exhibits left neglect and poor safety regarding his nonfunctional left hand. The OT fabricated a volar resting hand splint to help keep the client's joints in a safe, functional position. The client's wrist spasticity keeps causing the Velcro wrist strap to detach. Besides possibly fabricating a dorsal splint, which of the following is the best course of action for the OTA to remedy this problem?

    A. Remold the splint into a flexed wrist position

    B. Discontinue the splint

    C. Instruct the client to refasten the strap

    D. Use a D-ring and longer wrist strap

9. A primary purpose of an outrigger on a dynamic splint is:

    A. To ensure proper angle of pull

    B. To conform to the transverse and longitudinal arches

    C. To attach splint to the forearm

    D. To make the splint more durable

10. A child with cerebral palsy was issued a hand-based thumb spica splint last week to promote prehension. Today the child arrives with his mother and tells the OTA that the splint is uncomfortable due to it rubbing at the thumb IP joint, and he does not want to wear it. The OTA notices that the splint edge is rough and there is slight redness at the thumb IP. The OT has left for the day. Which of the following should the OTA do?

    A. Defer treatment and schedule an appointment with the OT tomorrow

    B. Fabricate a new splint

    C. Use a heat gun to smooth rough area

    D. Document that the child is making up excuses to avoid wearing the splint

Morreale, M. J. (2015). *Developing clinical competence: A workbook for the OTA.* Thorofare, NJ: SLACK Incorporated.

Worksheet 4-10

Splinting Instructions

You have just fabricated and issued a splint for a client who has osteoarthritis of her dominant thumb CMC joint. List at least eight things you need to educate the client about regarding the splint.

1.

2.

3.

4.

5.

6.

7.

8.

Morreale, M. J. (2015). *Developing clinical competence: A workbook for the OTA*. Thorofare, NJ: SLACK Incorporated.

Learning Activity 4-6: Custom Versus Prefabricated Splints

Choose a specific type of splint such as a resting hand splint, wrist extension splint, elbow extension splint, or dynamic MP extension splint. Make a list of all the materials and equipment needed to fabricate that splint. Use a professional catalog to calculate the exact cost of materials for making the splint, not including the practitioner's time or standard tools/equipment (i.e., heating unit, scissors, etc.). Also, determine if a similar prefabricated splint is available for purchase. Compare the cost of custom splint materials versus the price of the prefabricated splint. Which option would you choose for a client? Explain your rationale.

Name of splint _____

List several conditions this splint may be used for:_____

_____

_____

_____

Materials Required	Package Cost and Quantity	Unit Cost for One Splint
Example: Loop fastener	$25 per 25-foot roll	24 inches = $2.00

Equipment Required	Tools Required
Example: Electric splint pan	Example: Scissors

Total cost of splint (excluding labor costs): $_____

Prefabricated splint cost: $ _____

Rationale for Using a Custom Splint	Rationale for Using a Prefabricated Splint

Worksheet 4-11

Upper Extremity Safety

Stella is an 82-year-old client with a diagnosis of right CVA. Her left upper extremity is just beginning to exhibit some limited motor return in her shoulder and elbow, along with some active gross finger flexion. Stella also has poor left upper extremity sensation, homonymous hemianopsia, and moderate left neglect. When Stella sits in the wheelchair, she is unaware that her left arm tends to hang down over the side and get caught in the wheel. List six different preparatory or functional interventions that can improve the safety of Stella's upper extremity while she is sitting in her wheelchair. Determine the pros and cons of each method or task.

Intervention	Pros	Cons
1.		
2.		
3.		
4.		
5.		
6.		

Morreale, M. J. (2015). *Developing clinical competence: A workbook for the OTA.* Thorofare, NJ: SLACK Incorporated.

Answers to Worksheets

Occupational therapy practitioners must always use clinical judgment when selecting and implementing physical agent modalities, splints, therapeutic exercises, and other interventions. The OT and OTA must carefully consider multiple factors, such as the client's medical status and circumstances, precautions, contraindications, other available methods, evidence-based practice, and safety. Often, more than one type of physical agent, splint, exercise, or technique is used during a client's treatment program. Functional activities and occupations should always be incorporated into a client's intervention program. Worksheet answers contain general, sound guidelines, but may not be appropriate for all situations.

Worksheet 4-1: Therapeutic Exercises

Resources: Bandy & Sanders, 2008; Fairchild, 2013; Rybski, 2012

1. C. It will depend on the particular circumstances, but, in situations such as the one presented, a report of a minor complaint, such as "a little stretch" or "slight pull" is often not cause for major concern. However, if the client had a fragile wound, recent surgery such as a tendon or nerve repair, unstable joints, or reported a more severe complaint during ROM such as "severe pain" or "sharp pain," that would usually require more caution and a different line of thinking. Some other factors to consider are joint end feel and if a client's pain is new, different, unexpected, or disproportionate to the task at hand. Always keep in mind that pain may signify that something serious is happening, such as an infection, undiagnosed fracture, irritated nerve, or imminent risk of injury. For the situation depicted in this question, the OTA should not aggressively move or force the joint, but might gently try to hold the joint at point of slight tension for a brief hold (per client tolerance without creating severe pain) to see if the muscles relax and further ROM might be obtained. Many clients in occupational therapy have painful conditions that rehabilitation must gradually work through, but clinical judgment is always needed to ascertain what level of pain is or is not acceptable, expected, and safe and the appropriate techniques to apply.

2. D. The other answers all reflect inability to actively raise arm fully, which are indicators for self-ROM.

3. C. External rotation with the arm abducted is often a more difficult position for clients with shoulder conditions. The OTA can first try an alternate position, with shoulder adducted, to attempt gentle passive external rotation and determine if this will allow for safer, less painful, and improved ROM. However, realize caution must be taken with any report of severe or sharp pain. Clinical judgment is always needed to ascertain what level of pain is or is not acceptable, normal, and safe, depending on each client's diagnosis, precautions, and contraindications. Determine if a client's pain is new, different, unexpected, or disproportionate to the task at hand. Pain may signify that something serious is happening, such as an infection, undiagnosed fracture, irritated nerve, or reinjury. When in doubt, err on the side of caution and collaborate with your OT supervisor. In instances such as a healing fracture, tendon or nerve repair, or other joint conditions, further communication with the referring physician may be needed to determine healing status and how hard to "push" the client without risk of injury.

4. C. A tear or hole in an exercise band may cause it to break when it is pulled taut, possibly harming the client. The frequency of exercises and number of repetitions must be individualized for each client.

5. A. A shorter length will create more tension, thus needing more strength to pull band apart. Thera-Band resistance in order from weaker to stronger is yellow, red, green, blue (Hygenic Corp., 2008).

6. C. Constraint-induced movement therapy is not indicated for this client's diagnosis. Although he demonstrates some shoulder weakness, he still has functional use of his right upper extremity and no neurological deficit. He would benefit more from a strengthening program such as AAROM (active assistive) against gravity (answer C) and ADL modification. There are no noted joint restrictions or pain limiting AROM, so ultrasound and PROM are not needed at this time (although the client should be instructed in a home program of AROM to maintain mobility). PROM would also not be helpful for strengthening as it does not involve active muscle contractions. AROM on the table with a tabletop skateboard is in the gravity-minimized plane (needing only a muscle grade of poor) and would not really facilitate flexion of the shoulder. Functional activities should be incorporated and encouraged.

7. A. Finger to palm translation means manipulating an object to move it from the fingers into the palm. B, C, and D do not do that.

8. A. Isotonic contractions include eccentric and concentric contractions, which are occurring in the wrist flexors and extensors.

9. D. The biceps is actively shortening (as the elbow flexes) and lengthening (as the elbow extends) during the task.

10. D. Wrist extension during grasp and release is a typical mature pattern.

Worksheet 4-2: Open- and Closed-Kinetic-Chain Exercises

Closed-kinetic-chain exercises have a fixed end segment (such as in weight-bearing tasks), whereas open-kinetic-chain exercises have an end segment that is freely moveable (such as using dumbbells, exercise bands, reaching for objects, or holding items in space) (Gillen, 2011b; Wilk & Reinold, 2008). Open-kinetic-chain exercises may include resistive exercises that facilitate an isotonic, isometric, or isokinetic contraction (Bandy, 2008).

1. O. *Using exercise bands* to improve shoulder strength
2. O. *Turning a heavy jump rope* with another child holding the other end
3. C. *Weight bearing on forearm* while writing with the other hand
4. C. *Pushing a weighted toy shopping cart* while walking around an obstacle course
5. O. *Putting cans in upper kitchen cabinets*
6. O. *Using 1-lb. weights* to improve wrist strength
7. O. *Carrying a lunch tray* in the cafeteria
8. C. *Sanding* a wooden board using a sanding block
9. C. *Posing like a bear* with hands and feet on floor
10. O. *Using a reacher* to remove clothes from dryer
11. C. *Prone on elbows* while watching a wind-up toy move
12. C. *Rolling dough into piecrust shape using a rolling pin*
13. C. *Dynamic standing* when hanging clothes in closet
14. O. *Hanging clothes in closet* while standing
15. C. *Pressing/flattening therapy putty with palm* while standing at table
16. C. *Dynamic standing* while using a hula hoop
17. C. *Performing push-ups* against the wall while standing
18. O. *Moving rings from one side of an exercise arc to the other side*
19. C. *Applying lotion* to extremities
20. C. *Arm push-ups* while seated in preparation for transfers
21. O. *Cone stacking* to improve grip
22. O. *Waving a ribbon wand* to music
23. C. *Scrubbing a floor using a hand-held brush*
24. O. *Painting on an easel* while standing
25. C. *Sliding board transfer*

Worksheet 4-3: Preparatory Methods and Tasks

OTAs working in physical rehabilitation settings typically encounter clients who have impairment resulting from neurological conditions, such as CVA and traumatic brain injury. Traditional therapeutic approaches to facilitate motor control have included Bobath, Brunnstrom Movement Therapy, Rood, and Proprioceptive Neuromuscular Facilitation (Radomski & Latham, 2008). However, the evidence supports the use of newer approaches to motor learning, such as the task-oriented approach, which emphasizes functional interventions (Gillen, 2011a). Additional techniques, such as edema management or wound care, may be implemented to address other factors. It is very important to incorporate the client's affected upper extremity into functional tasks so that it is not just a passive appendage. The OTA can use techniques for motor learning such as constraint-induced movement therapy, bilateral activities, mental imagery, and occupation-based activities that facilitate motor skills (Gillen, 2011a, 2011b). While adhering to any precautions and contraindications regarding the client's present situation (such as fracture-healing status and postoperative protocols), the OTA should use a function-based approach as much as possible to promote awareness of the involved side, maintain mobility, and improve occupational performance (Gillen, 2011a; Morawski & Padilla, 2012).

1. A. Vibration may be used for scar management or, according to Rood's facilitation principles, the recruitment of muscle fibers (Bentzel, 2008; Rust, 2008). It is not a standard intervention for edema management.

2. B. Eye-hand coordination is not a typical deficit associated with carpal tunnel syndrome or release, although fine-motor skills may be affected due to weakness or sensory deficits (Eaton, n.d.). Median nerve compression may affect strength of the intrinsic muscles in the thenar eminence that controls thumb MP flexion, palmar abduction, and opposition, thus affecting tip pinch. Thumb adduction (used in lateral pinch) is ulnar nerve innervated, so that is not the best answer; although diminished thumb sensation could hinder lateral pinch. The hypothenar muscles (on ulnar side of hand) are intrinsic muscles innervated by the ulnar nerve and involve the small finger.

3. B. Wounds are classified as red (healing granulation tissue), yellow (has exudate such as pus), or black (necrotic tissue) (Bracciano, 2008; Evans & McAuliffe, 2002). Answers C and D actually indicate an increase in wound size.

4. C. Although all the exercises indicated are appropriate, it is best to not use exercise putty directly over clothing, as putty may stick to it and possibly ruin clothing.

5. D. The child's feet need to be supported for trunk stability. It is not productive for the child to write with the nondominant hand. The affected hand should be positioned with forearm in pronation resting on table for weight bearing to help inhibit tone and provide postural stability (Levit, 2008).

6. B. The OTA should have the clinical skill to perform stump wrapping. The appropriate method is a figure-8 diagonal application (Stubblefield & Armstrong, 2008).

7. C. Practitioners specially trained in the Wilbarger protocol use a specific type of brush and special techniques to apply deep pressure and proprioception to a child's limbs and back to help reduce sensory defensiveness (Wilbarger & Wilbarger, 2002). If the arm was simply being cleaned, the OTA would be using soap and water.

8. A. Due to its anatomic architecture, the hand should not be completely flattened and the OTA should take care to maintain arches of the hand (Levit, 2008; Morawski & Padilla, 2012). A weak upper extremity may cause the elbow to buckle, which is unsafe. Gradual weight shifting/leaning toward the affected side will help to promote weight bearing through that affected extremity so that it can provide stability during functional tasks. Weight shift toward the unaffected side is also useful to lengthen muscles of a weak arm and trunk (Levit, 2008). A function-based approach should be used to incorporate the involved extremity in weight-bearing activities for daily occupations, such as stabilizing objects, wiping a table, using extremity as a postural support while dressing, etc. (Gillen, 2011b).

9. D. The arm must move away from the body to have tension in the exercise band for external rotation. Standing with the right side closest to doorknob would not allow for tension in the band.

10. C. A client needing a wheelchair should be assessed to ensure proper fit, adequate support, optimal positioning, and to determine the specific type of seat cushion or adaptations that may be indicated. Seat width (not depth) should provide slight clearance (1.5 to 2 inches) between the client's hips and the side panels of wheelchair to avoid skin breakdown at trochanters. Seat depth should allow for approximately 2 inches of clearance between the edge of seat and popliteal space (back of knees). Armrest height is normally measured with elbow placed at 90 degrees. Wheelchair back height generally should be slightly below the inferior angles of the scapula, although some clients may need a higher back for greater trunk support or a lower back to allow for greater propulsion (Fairchild, 2013; Minor & Minor, 2006).

Worksheet 4-4: Physical Agent Modality Categories

Indicate the pertinent category for each of the physical agent modalities listed below (AOTA, 2012; Bracciano, 2008).

	Physical Agent Modality	*Superficial Thermal Agent*	*Deep Thermal Agent*	*Electrotherapeutic Agent*	*Mechanical Device*
1.	Fluidotherapy	*			
2.	Transcutaneous electrical nerve stimulation (TENS)			*	
3.	Iontophoresis			*	

	Physical Agent Modality	Superficial Thermal Agent	Deep Thermal Agent	Electrotherapeutic Agent	Mechanical Device
4.	Hot pack	*			
5.	Ultrasound		*		
6.	Whirlpool	*			
7.	Vasopneumatic device				*
8.	Cryotherapy	*			
9.	Neuromuscular electrical stimulation (NMES)			*	
10	Functional electrical stimulation (FES)			*	
11.	Continuous passive motion (CPM)				*
12.	Paraffin	*			
13.	High-voltage pulsed current (HVPC)			*	
14.	Cold pack	*			
15.	Hydrotherapy	*			
16.	Phonophoresis		*		
17.	Short-wave diathermy		*		
18.	Vapocoolant spray	*			
19.	Infrared	*			
20.	Lymphedema pump				*

Worksheet 4-5: Selecting Physical Agent Modalities

Resources: Bracciano, 2008; Cameron, 2009; Knight & Draper, 2008
1. H. Acute PIP hyperextension injury with pain and edema (cold pack)
2. I. Shoulder stiffness due to rheumatoid arthritis (hot pack)
3. L. Muscle reeducation to learn how to minimize involuntary upper trapezius muscle contraction (biofeedback)
4. D. Healed carpal tunnel release with stiffness, fair light touch sensation, intact protective sensation, and scar hypersensitivity (Fluidotherapy)
   The moving particles can be used to reduce hypersensitivity and the modality temperature can be lowered to avoid harm due to client's slightly decreased sensation.
5. J. Thumb CMC arthritis with pain and stiffness (paraffin)
6. E. Manage edema following soft tissue trauma (vasopneumatic pump)
7. A. Open wound requiring debridement (whirlpool)
8. F. Chronic biceps pain upon discharge from occupational therapy (TENS)
9. B. Conditions requiring mechanical PROM (CPM)
10. K. Lateral epicondylitis requiring topical medication delivery through the skin (iontophoresis)
11. G. CVA with hemiparesis and shoulder subluxation (NMES)
12. C. PIP joint contracture and scar adhesions following a healed laceration to volar index finger (ultrasound)
    Ultrasound can provide thermal and nonthermal effects to promote tissue changes and healing.

Worksheet 4-6: Using Physical Agent Modalities Safely

Resources: Bracciano, 2008; Cameron, 2009; Knight & Draper, 2008
1. C. Paraffin is contraindicated for areas containing open wounds, severe edema, or poor sensation. Superficial heat is used to decrease stiffness and facilitate tendon gliding.
2. D. The hot pack is used on the client's shoulder, so there is no need to remove jewelry from wrist and hand. An anti-static mat or plastic bag is not indicated for this modality.

3. C. The client is at risk for a burn, so the hot pack should be removed before the OTA spends time looking for the OT. The hydrocollator temperature should be checked before a hot pack is placed on a client.

4. B. Due to how an extremity must be placed in the Fluidotherapy unit, this modality is not appropriate for shoulder use. Heat should not be applied to a rheumatic joint that is acutely inflamed.

5. D. Cryotherapy is use of a cold thermal agent. A frozen gel pack requires a cover when placed on the skin. It is important to monitor what stage the client is feeling from a gel or ice pack, as the client generally experiences a progression of effects. Realize the client is at risk for tissue damage if cold is administered for an extended time or on areas with absent sensation (insensate).

6. B. Care should be taken to protect the client's neck from the hot pack possibly touching it. Clients should not lie directly on a hot pack as pressure on the pack, oozing gel, or excess water may result in a burn.

7. B. Clients should wash and dry hands before a paraffin treatment. A plastic bag is normally placed over the client's hand **after** the hand has been dipped in paraffin. The client's affected hand should typically remain still during paraffin dips to avoid breaking the paraffin "glove," which would allow hot wax to seep underneath and possibly burn the skin. The client should not touch the bottom or sides of the unit as these areas could possibly be very hot, causing a burn.

8. C. It is contraindicated to apply heat to a burn. Most likely there is no need to contact the client's physician for simple sunburn unless the client is exhibiting other adverse effects such as dehydration, sunstroke, infection, skin rash, or hives. The client should be able to work on other aspects of the intervention plan, such as functional activities.

9. D. Heat modalities and ultrasound are contraindicated for malignant areas.

10. A. Cold is beneficial to reduce acute inflammation but is contraindicated for clients with cold intolerance and poor circulation. Heat, rather than cold, helps to improve soft tissue extensibility. The carpal tunnel release should be well healed by this time and there is no indication of resulting sensory deficits.

Worksheet 4-7: Physical Agent Modality Basics

Resources: Bracciano, 2008; Cameron, 2009; Knight & Draper, 2008

1. A. The use of PAMs alone is not considered occupational therapy (AOTA, 2012).
2. C.
3. C.
4. D.
5. A. Ultrasound and TENS are not superficial thermal agents, so the OTA cannot use them in that particular state.
6. A. Fluidotherapy can be used for both desensitization and AROM and the unit temperature can be lowered to minimize heating effect as necessary.
7. D. An OT must have service competency regarding a modality in order to supervise an OTA administering that modality (AOTA, 2012). If the client needs a modality that the OT is not competent to supervise, the client should be referred to another practitioner. (PRN stands for "as needed.")
8. D. The OTA should only implement the modalities contained in the OT's intervention plan. However, the OTA may document what the client said and then speak to the OT to determine if the treatment plan should be modified to include paraffin.
9. B. Superficial heat is used to decrease pain, relax muscles, and improve tissue extensibility in preparation for therapeutic exercises/activities. Cold may be used following exercises/activities to prevent flare up of the condition. It is usually not indicated to implement both hot packs and paraffin to the same area during a single session.
10. C. Used wax should always be discarded to help keep the paraffin unit clean. Paraffin completely hardens so it will not be useful for exercises at home.

Worksheet 4-8: Selecting Splint Interventions

Resources: Coppard & Lohman, 2008; Jacobs & Austin, 2003

1. K. Carpal tunnel syndrome *(volar wrist cock-up splint)*
2. M. Boutonniere deformity ring finger *(PIP extension splint)*

3. R. Upper extremity amputation *(body-powered prosthesis)*

4. P. Small finger metacarpal fracture *(ulnar gutter splint)*

5. N. Dupuytren's release *(forearm-based dorsal extension splint)*

6. T. C6-C7 spinal cord injury *(tenodesis splint)*

7. F. Flexor tendon repair of digits *(dorsal blocking splint)*

8. C. Brachial plexus injury *(airplane splint [shoulder abduction splint])*

9. H. Swan neck deformity *(figure-8 finger splint [PIP hyperextension block splint])*

10. O. Mallet finger *(DIP extension splint)*

11. B. Low level ulnar nerve injury *(MP extension blocking splint)*

12. A. Burns to hand/wrist *(resting hand splint)*

13. S. Extrinsic extensor tightness of digits *(composite flexion splint)*

14. G. De Quervain's tenosynovitis *(forearm-based thumb spica splint [long opponens splint])*

15. L. Elbow flexion contracture *(anterior elbow splint)*

16. J. MP joints requiring realignment secondary to rheumatoid arthritis *(ulnar deviation splint)*

17. D. Flexed digits of a client with end-stage dementia causing skin breakdown in hand *(palm protector, can also use a soft hand cone)*

18. E. Low level median nerve injury *(short opponens splint)*

19. Q. Lateral epicondylitis *(counterforce brace [tennis elbow strap])*

20. I. Radial nerve palsy *(dynamic MP extension splint)*

Worksheet 4-9: Splinting Basics

Resources: Coppard & Lohman, 2008; Jacobs & Austin, 2003

1. C. A volar wrist extension splint begins proximal to the MPs and continues two-thirds the length of the forearm. A potential pressure area is the ulnar styloid.

2. C. The OTA should not discontinue the splint without physician approval and the OT's collaboration, particularly for an unhealed fracture.

3. B. While a pattern may be placed in the client's chart for future reference, it is not necessary to do so. Patterns are usually traced onto the thermoplastic material so that will not avoid marks. Making a pattern does help prevent costly mistakes by not using a trial and error approach. However, the primary purpose of a pattern is to help ensure proper splint size and fit, determine best design, and fabricate the splint more efficiently.

4. D. Never place a splint from the heating source directly onto the client, as the high heat could cause a skin burn. Cooling times vary by type and thickness of material.

5. A. The splint should position the thumb in a functional position.

6. A. A mallet finger splint typically only immobilizes the DIP joint.

7. A. Splint generally should be two-thirds the length of the forearm.

8. D. Looping the strap through a D-ring and creating more hook and loop fastener contact will increase stability. This should be considered before fabricating a new splint. However, it is essential to ensure that this new strap configuration does not cause any harmful pressure on the client's wrist. While answer C would work, it is only a temporary solution and not the best option.

9. A. Dynamic splints require outriggers carefully placed to allow a proper angle of pull (normally 90 degrees), to avoid traction or compression of a joint.

10. C. The OTA should be able to easily modify the splint with a heat gun (to smooth the rough edge) so the splint is better tolerated by the child. The OTA's observation of redness indicates the child is not simply making up an excuse. Education should be provided to the parent and child regarding precautions and monitoring of skin integrity. A follow-up splint check should be scheduled and the OT also notified.

Worksheet 4-10: Splinting Instructions

1. Purpose of splint
2. Wearing schedule
3. How to don and doff splint
4. Home exercise program to prevent stiffness of immobilized joints
5. Care and cleaning of splint
6. Skin integrity (keeping skin dry, check for pressure areas)
7. Possible problems that may arise (pressure areas, pain, edema, etc.)
8. Splint protection (keep splint away from heat sources, do not leave in car on hot day)
9. Contact information if problems should arise
10. Follow-up appointment (bring splint)

Worksheet 4-11: Upper Extremity Safety

While proper body alignment is essential, it is also very important to incorporate the client's involved upper extremity into functional tasks as much as possible so that it is not just a passive appendage. For clients with CVA, the OTA can use various techniques such as weight bearing, guiding, bilateral activities, constraint-induced movement therapy, task-oriented reaching, etc., incorporated into occupations to facilitate functional motor skills at appropriate stages of recovery (Gillen, 2011a, 2011b). The inclusion of the client's affected extremity in everyday tasks helps to promote awareness of that side, maintain mobility, and improve its function (Gillen, 2011a, 2011b; Morawski & Padilla, 2012). Of course, any precautions or contraindications must always be adhered to (i.e., fracture, fragile wound, etc.). Occupational therapy practitioners must always consider the current evidence, the pros and cons of each intervention method for a specific client, and then choose a method or combination of methods most appropriate for the particular situation.

Intervention	*Pros*	*Cons*
Support left upper extremity on a lap tray	• Safer position for left upper extremity • Decreased potential for injury • Left upper extremity in visual field • May improve trunk upright posture	• May be considered a restraint • Arm may slide off lap tray • Potential for skin breakdown • Passive position
Support left upper extremity on an arm trough/arm support	• Safer position for left upper extremity • Decreased potential for injury • Left upper extremity may be in visual field • May improve trunk upright posture	• Arm may slide off of arm trough/support • May not be a naturally comfortable position for client's upper extremity • Potential for skin breakdown • Passive position
Educate client on proper position of left upper extremity and risk of injury. Provide verbal and written reminders. Encourage client to self-correct arm position with unaffected hand.	• Increases client awareness of problem and self-correction of problem	• Unilateral neglect or cognitive deficits may interfere with carryover • Client may not be able to reach and position extremity with unaffected hand

Intervention	Pros	Cons
Provide sling for left upper extremity	• Keeps arm from getting caught in wheel	• Places arm in a nonfunctional, passive position • May lead to contracture for shoulder adduction and internal rotation • Arm may slide out of sling • May cause pressure around neck • Impedes voluntary motion
Have client look in mirror and determine what is problematic with her wheelchair posture	• Increases client awareness of problem and self-correction of problem	• Unilateral neglect or cognitive deficits may interfere with carryover
Use bilateral techniques and active involvement of involved arm to incorporate the extremity in functional task performance	• Increases client awareness of extremity • Promotes functional movement patterns and motor learning for occupations • Assists in joint mobility • Helps prevent disuse	• Client may overstretch joints or may drop the arm and cause injury if too aggressive, inattentive, or not careful • Unilateral neglect or cognitive deficits may interfere with carryover
Other:		

References

Accreditation Council for Occupational Therapy Education. (2012). 2011 Accreditation Council for Occupational Therapy Education (ACOTE) standards. *American Journal of Occupational Therapy, 66*(6 Suppl.), S6-S74. doi: 10.5014/ajot.2012.66S6

American Occupational Therapy Association. (2012). Physical agent modalities. *American Journal of Occupational Therapy, 66*(6 Suppl.), S78-S80. doi: 10.5014/ajot.2012.66S78

American Occupational Therapy Association. (2014). Occupational therapy practice framework: Domain and process (3rd ed.). *American Journal of Occupational Therapy, 68*(1 Suppl.), S1-S48. doi: 10.5014/ajot.2014.682006

Bandy, W. D. (2008). Open-chain-resistance training. In W. D. Bandy & B. Sanders (Eds.), *Therapeutic exercise for physical therapist assistants: Techniques for intervention* (2nd ed.) (pp. 103-136). Baltimore, MD: Lippincott Williams & Wilkins.

Bandy, W. D., & Sanders, B. (2008). *Therapeutic exercise for physical therapist assistants: Techniques for intervention* (2nd ed.). Baltimore, MD: Lippincott Williams & Wilkins.

Bentzel, K. (2008). Optimizing sensory abilities and capacities. In M. V. Radomski & C. A. T. Latham (Eds.), *Occupational therapy for physical dysfunction* (6th ed.) (pp. 714-727). Baltimore, MD: Lippincott Williams & Wilkins.

Bracciano, A. G. (2008). *Physical agent modalities: Theory and application for the occupational therapist* (2nd ed.). Thorofare, NJ: SLACK Incorporated.

Cameron, M. H. (2009). *Physical agents in rehabilitation: From research to practice* (3rd ed.). St. Louis, MO: Saunders.

Coppard, B. M., & Lohman, H. (Eds.). (2008). *Splinting: A clinical reasoning and problem-solving approach* (3rd ed.). St. Louis, MO: Mosby.

Eaton, C. (n.d.). *The electronic textbook of hand surgery: Carpal tunnel syndrome.* Retrieved from www.eatonhand.com/hw/hw006.htm

Evans, R. B., & McAuliffe, J. A. (2002). Wound classification and management. In E. J. Mackin, A. D. Callahan, T. M. Skirven, L. H. Schneider, & A. L. Osterman (Eds.), *Rehabilitation of the hand and upper extremity* (5th ed.) (pp. 311-330). St. Louis, MO: Mosby.

Fairchild, S. L. (2013). *Pierson and Fairchild's principles & techniques of patient care* (5th ed.). St. Louis, MO: Saunders.

Gillen, G. (Ed.). (2011a). *Stroke rehabilitation: A function-based approach* (3rd ed.). St. Louis, MO: Elsevier Mosby.

Gillen, G. (2011b). Upper extremity function and management. In G. Gillen (Ed.), *Stroke rehabilitation: A function-based approach* (3rd ed.) (pp. 218-279). St. Louis, MO: Elsevier Mosby.

Hygenic Corp. (2008). *Thera-Band exercise bands.* Retrieved from www.thera-band.com/store/products.php?ProductID=26

Jacobs, M. A., & Austin, N. M. (Eds.). (2003). *Splinting the hand and upper extremity: Principles and process.* Baltimore, MD: Lippincott Williams & Wilkins.

Knight, K. L., & Draper, D. O. (2008). *Therapeutic modalities: The art and science.* Baltimore, MD: Lippincott Williams & Wilkins.

Levit, K. (2008). Optimizing motor behavior using the Bobath approach. In M. V. Radomski, & C. A. T. Latham (Eds.), *Occupational therapy for physical dysfunction* (6th ed.) (pp. 642-666). Baltimore, MD: Lippincott Williams & Wilkins.

Minor, M. A., & Minor, S. D. (2006). *Patient care skills* (5th ed.). Upper Saddle River, NJ: Pearson Education, Inc.

Morawski, D. L., & Padilla, R. (2012). Working with elders who have had cerebrovascular accidents. In R. L. Padilla, S. Byers-Connon, & H. L. Lohman (Eds.), *Occupational therapy with elders: Strategies for the COTA* (3rd ed.) (pp. 263-274). Maryland Heights, MO: Elsevier Mosby.

Radomski, M. V., & Latham, C. A. T. (Eds.). (2008). *Occupational therapy for physical dysfunction* (6th ed.). Baltimore, MD: Lippincott Williams & Wilkins.

Rust, K. L. (2008). Managing deficit of first-level motor control capacities using Rood and proprioceptive neuromuscular facilitation techniques. In M. V. Radomski, & C. A. T. Latham (Eds.), *Occupational therapy for physical dysfunction* (6th ed.) (pp. 691-713). Baltimore, MD: Lippincott Williams & Wilkins.

Rybski, M. F. (2012). *Kinesiology for occupational therapy* (2nd ed.). Thorofare, NJ: SLACK Incorporated.

Stubblefield, K., & Armstrong, A. (2008). Amputations and prosthetics. In M. V. Radomski, & C. A. T. Latham (Eds.), *Occupational therapy for physical dysfunction* (6th ed.) (pp. 1264-1294). Baltimore, MD: Lippincott Williams & Wilkins.

Wilbarger, J., & Wilbarger, P. (2002). The Wilbarger approach to treating sensory defensiveness. In A. C. Bundy, S. L. Lane, & E. A. Murray (Eds.), *Sensory integration theory and practice* (2nd ed.) (pp. 335-338). Philadelphia, PA: F. A. Davis.

Wilk, K. E., & Reinold, M. M. (2008). Closed-kinetic-chain exercise. In W. D. Bandy & B. Sanders (Eds.), *Therapeutic exercise for physical therapist assistants: Techniques for intervention* (2nd ed.) (pp. 171-188). Baltimore, MD: Lippincott Williams & Wilkins.

Chapter 5

Incorporating Activities and Occupations

Occupational therapy practitioners use a variety of methods and interventions to facilitate occupational performance and role competence, maintain health and wellness, and improve quality of life (American Occupational Therapy Association [AOTA], 2014). Depending on the client's unique circumstances, the intervention plan may include approaches such as developing or remediating specific client factors and performance skills; modifying the task, environment, or performance patterns; or compensating for lost function (AOTA, 2014). As noted in Chapter 4, although preparatory interventions can be an important part of a client's intervention plan, these methods and tasks should supplement, but never replace, activities and occupations (AOTA, 2014). Occupational therapy practitioners must use a holistic approach that incorporates meaningful "real-life" interventions that address or support the client's therapeutic goals for occupational engagement (AOTA, 2014). Activities and occupations are emphasized in this chapter, along with select preparatory methods and tasks that also contribute to occupational performance (i.e., client/family education and training, provision of adaptive/durable medical equipment (DME), therapeutic exercises, etc.). Note that space limitations allow for only select initial evaluation data to be presented here. A "real" evaluation would include more complete information, such as the specific aspects of occupations needing assistance and the various factors, contexts, or performance skills hindering or supporting occupational performance. Answers to worksheet exercises are provided at the end of the chapter.

Contents

Morreale, M. J.
Developing Clinical Competence: A Workbook for the OTA (pp. 137-175).
© 2015 SLACK Incorporated.

Worksheet 5-1

Teaching-Learning Process (Total Hip Replacement)

Elaine, a client in acute care, is a 65-year-old female who had left total hip replacement surgery (posterolateral approach) 2 days ago. She presently has non-weight-bearing status for her affected leg, and her secondary diagnoses include hypertension and hyperlipidemia. Elaine was evaluated by the OT yesterday and received preliminary instruction in total hip precautions. Upon reviewing the initial evaluation report, the OTA notes that the client's upper extremity function and cognition are intact, but the client requires moderate assistance to transfer using a walker. The expected discharge plan is for Elaine to go to a short-term rehabilitation facility 3 days from now and then eventually return home. Today the OTA was delegated the task of teaching the client lower body dressing techniques. Consider the process for implementing this intervention session, such as equipment/supplies needed, methods of instruction, and sequence of steps that the OTA should use for the occupation of dressing.

1. Where will the session take place? _____

2. What is the anticipated length of session? _____

3. What equipment/supplies will the OTA need to bring to the session? _____
    _____
    _____

4. What are several things the OTA should do prior to entering the client's room?_____
    _____
    _____
    _____

5. List the general steps of how the session should be implemented:

    A. Perform hand hygiene and use _____ as indicated

    B. Introduce OTA and explain _____

    C. _____
        _____
        _____

    D. _____
        _____
        _____

    E. _____
        _____
        _____

    F. _____
        _____
        _____

    G. _____
        _____
        _____

    H. _____
        _____
        _____

    I. _____
        _____
        _____

Worksheet 5-1 (continued)

Teaching-Learning Process (Total Hip Replacement)

J. _____

K. _____

L. _____

M. _____

N. _____

O. _____

P. _____

In what ways, if any, would you implement the intervention session any differently if the client were 90 years old?

Learning Activity 5-1: Teaching-Learning Process (Carpal Tunnel Syndrome)

Your client, Ben, is a 35-year-old computer programmer diagnosed with carpal tunnel syndrome in his dominant right hand. He is otherwise in good health. Ben was evaluated by the OT at an outpatient clinic 3 days ago. Here is some information taken from the initial evaluation report:

- *Chief complaint:* Ben reports he has been experiencing decreased hand strength and increased pain, numbness, and tingling in his right thumb, index, and long fingers for the past 4 months.
- *Pain:* Right hand reported as 7/10.
- *Sensation:* Right hand: Two-point discrimination: 8-mm index and long fingers, 5-mm ring and small fingers. Phalen's test is positive, eliciting numbness/tingling at 15 seconds.
- *Active range of motion (AROM):* Both upper extremities within normal limits (WNL)
- *BADL/IADL:* Ben's symptoms are creating difficulty with sleeping, job performance, his daily exercise routine at the gym, and yard maintenance.

Strength	Right Hand	Left Hand
Grip	78 lbs.	98 lbs.
3-point pinch	20 lbs.	28 lbs.
Lateral pinch	28 lbs.	30 lbs.
Tip pinch	17 lbs.	22 lbs.

After completing Ben's evaluation, the OT fabricated and issued a volar wrist immobilization splint for Ben to wear at work, nighttime, and during heavy tasks. Today Ben has his first follow-up appointment, and the OTA will be working with Ben to start teaching him median nerve gliding exercises, tendon gliding exercises, and ergonomics for work. Consider the process for implementing these interventions, such as equipment/supplies needed, specific methods of instruction, and sequence of steps that the OTA should follow. Incorporate several activities needed for Ben's desired level of job performance.

1. Where will the session take place? _____

2. What is the anticipated length of session? _____

3. What equipment/supplies will the OTA need to gather for the therapy session? _____

   _____

   _____

4. Use resources to locate specific instructions/pictures for the nerve and tendon gliding exercises and ergonomic recommendations that Ben will need to be instructed on.

5. The OTA has collaborated with the OT and reviewed Ben's chart. List the general sequence of how the OTA should implement all of Ben's interventions for today, including several activities needed for his job:

   A. Perform hand hygiene

   B. Introduce OTA and explain _____

   _____

   _____

   C. _____

   _____

   _____

   _____

   D. _____

   _____

   _____

E. _____
_____
_____

F. _____
_____
_____

G. _____
_____
_____

H. _____
_____
_____

I. _____
_____
_____

J. _____
_____
_____

K. _____
_____
_____

L. _____
_____
_____

M. _____
_____
_____

N. _____
_____
_____

How do the tendon and nerve gliding exercises relate to Ben's occupational performance?

Worksheet 5-2

Cerebrovascular Accident Interventions

Marvin, a 62-year-old male diagnosed with a cerebrovascular accident (CVA), was just admitted to a subacute rehabilitation facility. Marvin retired from his postal worker job 2 years ago, got divorced last year, and lived alone independently prior to his stroke. Here is some information taken from Marvin's occupational therapy initial evaluation report:

Upper extremity status:
- Hand dominance: Right
- ROM: Passive range of motion (PROM) WNL both upper extremities
- Strength: Right upper extremity flaccid, left upper extremity within functional limits (WFL)
- Sensation: Intact protective sensation right upper extremity

Communication: Demonstrates dysarthria, but understands and follows three-step verbal commands.

Balance and mobility: Weakness noted in trunk and right lower extremity. Dynamic sitting and standing balance are fair. While seated in wheelchair, client tends to lean to the right and slide forward with a posterior pelvic tilt. He requires moderate assistance to ambulate using mobility device.

BADL: Requires moderate assistance for self-care and transfers.

In collaboration with the OT, which of the following equipment, adaptive devices, or modalities are likely appropriate for an OTA to use with Marvin at this time to address his primary deficits? Assume that interventions would include not only the provision of a particular piece of equipment or DME, but actual instruction and practice in its use. Mark Y (yes) or N (no).

1. _____ Rocker knife

2. _____ Non-slip matting

3. _____ Built-up utensils

4. _____ Plate guard

5. _____ Walker

6. _____ Power wheelchair

7. _____ Electric razor

8. _____ Sock aid

9. _____ Therapy putty

10. _____ Exercise bands

11. _____ Pulleys

12. _____ Vest restraint

13. _____ Wheelchair arm support

14. _____ Soap-on-a-rope

15. _____ Wash mitt

Morreale, M. J. (2015). *Developing clinical competence: A workbook for the OTA*. Thorofare, NJ: SLACK Incorporated.

Worksheet 5-2 (continued)

Cerebrovascular Accident Interventions

16. _____ Soap/shampoo dispenser

17. _____ Long-handled sponge

18. _____ Tub seat/bench

19. _____ Hot pack to right shoulder

20. _____ Paraffin to right hand

21. _____ Constraint-induced movement therapy

22. _____ Teach self-ROM

23. _____ Lapboard

24. _____ Large pegboard

25. _____ Nine-Hole Peg Test

Worksheet 5-3

Total Hip Replacement Interventions

Anna is a 74-year-old female who had left hip replacement surgery (posterolateral approach) 5 days ago due to degenerative joint disease that was causing severe left hip pain. She was admitted to a skilled nursing facility yesterday for short-term rehabilitation, with an expected discharge plan to return home in several weeks. Anna's medical history includes hypertension, type 2 diabetes, and Vitamin B_{12} deficiency. She never married, retired from her teaching job at age 62, and has lived alone independently in a senior citizen apartment for the past 9 years. Doctor's orders state that Anna is not yet allowed to bear any weight on her left lower extremity. Anna presently requires minimal assistance to transfer and ambulate short distances and is unable to perform lower body dressing and bathing due to her total hip precautions. Both upper extremities exhibit good ROM and muscle strength of fair plus. The intervention plan for Anna includes goals for modified independence in lower body bathing, dressing, and transfers, and also to increase upper extremity muscle strength by half a muscle grade to support ADL independence. In collaboration with the OT, which of the following equipment, adaptive devices, or techniques are likely appropriate for an OTA to use with Anna at this time to address her primary deficits? Assume that interventions would include not only the provision of a particular piece of equipment or DME, but actual instruction and practice in its use. Mark Y (yes) or N (no).

1. _____ Raised toilet seat

2. _____ Adduction cushion

3. _____ Built-up utensils

4. _____ Commode

5. _____ Crossing legs to tie shoes

6. _____ Walker

7. _____ Power wheelchair

8. _____ Long-handled shoehorn

9. _____ Sock aid

10. _____ Hot pack to left hip

11. _____ Paraffin to left hand

12. _____ Teach stair climbing with crutches

13. _____ Wheelchair arm support

14. _____ Exercise bands

15. _____ Quad cane

16. _____ Elastic shoelaces

17. _____ Wedge cushion for wheelchair

18. _____ Reacher

Morreale, M. J. (2015). *Developing clinical competence: A workbook for the OTA*. Thorofare, NJ: SLACK Incorporated.

Worksheet 5-3 (continued)

Total Hip Replacement Interventions

19. _____ Long-handled sponge

20. _____ Tub seat/bench

21. _____ Leg lifter

22. _____ Constraint-induced movement therapy

23. _____ Sliding board

24. _____ Buttonhook

25. _____ Hospital bed for home

Worksheet 5-4

Improving Basic and Instrumental Activities of Daily Living Occupations

1. An OTA is working with a client on functional ambulation in the kitchen so that the client can prepare meals safely. The client uses a walker due to a left femur fracture and partial weight-bearing status. Which of the following is the correct sequence for using the walker?

   A. Advance walker, then weak leg, then strong leg

   B. Advance weak leg, then walker, then strong leg

   C. Advance walker, then strong leg, then weak leg

   D. Advance strong leg, then weak leg, then walker

2. A client admitted to an inpatient rehabilitation hospital has a diagnosis of bilateral below-knee amputations and is not a candidate for prostheses. He is independent in sliding board transfers, but his wheelchair will not be able to fit through his bathroom doorway at his small, ranch-style home. The OTA should instruct the client in use of which of the following to enable him to perform toileting independently at home?

   A. Raised toilet seat and grab bar

   B. Commode

   C. Power mobility scooter

   D. Platform walker

3. An OTA is working on transfer training with a client who uses a walker and is diagnosed with Parkinson's disease. When having the client transfer from a chair to a standing position, the OTA should instruct the client to do which of the following?

   A. Keep client's knees close together

   B. Hold onto a transfer belt around the OTA's waist

   C. Lean forward over client's center of gravity

   D. Have client use his arms to push up from walker

4. A client in acute care is diagnosed with a right CVA. His left upper extremity is flaccid and he exhibits fair dynamic standing balance, left neglect, and impulsivity. One of the client's goals is to achieve independence in shaving. Which of the following would best facilitate the client's shaving performance?

   A. Sitting on edge of bed using a bedside table (with mirror) and a safety razor

   B. Standing at sink using electric razor

   C. Sitting in a chair at the sink using electric razor

   D. Sitting in a chair at the sink using a safety razor

5. A client diagnosed with amyotrophic lateral sclerosis is working with an OTA to improve self-feeding skills. The client has good trunk control, but exhibits weakness of the intrinsic hand muscles and oral musculature. To best facilitate feeding skills, the OTA should place the client in which of the following positions?

   A. Sitting in a chair and using an electronic feeding device

   B. Sitting in a chair with chin slightly tucked

   C. Sitting in a chair with neck hyperextended

   D. Sitting in a chair with client's pelvis in a posterior tilt

Worksheet 5-4 (continued)

Improving Basic and Instrumental Activities of Daily Living Occupations

6. A 5-year-old child with a developmental delay is having difficulty donning a coat due to motor planning difficulties with bringing the coat around her back. Which primary method would best help the child become independent in donning her coat?

    A. Use an over-the-head method to don coat

    B. Use mirroring technique

    C. Write down step-by-step instructions

    D. Use a larger size coat

7. An OTA is teaching energy conservation techniques to a female client who has a diagnosis of chronic obstructive pulmonary disease (COPD), uses portable oxygen, and fatigues easily. The client is able to ambulate short distances using a rolling walker. Which of the following instructions would be most useful for homemaking?

    A. Use a barbecue grill instead of having to bend when using the oven broiler

    B. Use a tub seat when bathing

    C. Exhale before picking up a laundry basket, then inhale while placing it on top of dryer

    D. Use a flat sheet rather than a fitted sheet

8. An OTA is working with a client who is diagnosed with a complete C4 spinal cord injury. Assuming the OTA is competent in all the tasks below, which of the following would be the least appropriate occupational therapy intervention for this client?

    A. Instruct client in use of a mouthstick to operate computer keyboard

    B. Instruct client in functional mobility using a sip-and-puff wheelchair

    C. Instruct client in use of environmental controls to operate TV

    D. Instruct client in use of hand controls for driving

9. An OTA is working with a male client who is diagnosed with a complete C6 spinal cord injury. Which of the following would be the least appropriate occupational therapy intervention for this client?

    A. Instruct client in use of a buttonhook

    B. Instruct client in adaptive shaving techniques

    C. Instruct client in use of a wrist-driven hinge orthosis for feeding

    D. Instruct client in wheelchair push-ups to relieve pressure while sitting

10. An OTA is working with a client who is diagnosed with a complete C7-C8 spinal cord injury. Which of the following would be the least appropriate OT intervention for this client?

    A. Instruct client in light meal preparation

    B. Instruct client in functional mobility using a power wheelchair

    C. Instruct client in wheelchair push-ups to relieve pressure while sitting

    D. Instruct client in use of a padded bench/chair for bathing

Morreale, M. J. (2015). *Developing clinical competence: A workbook for the OTA*. Thorofare, NJ: SLACK Incorporated.

Worksheet 5-5

Total Knee Replacement Interventions

Harvey is a 70-year-old male who had right knee replacement surgery 3 days ago and was subsequently admitted to a subacute rehabilitation facility yesterday. Harvey lives with his wife in a senior citizen apartment building with elevator access. Prior to admission, he worked part-time as a sales clerk in a home improvement store and was independent in all ADL, including driving. Expected discharge to home is in 1 week. Here is some information taken from Harvey's occupational therapy evaluation report:

Weight-bearing status: Partial weight bearing right lower extremity

ROM: Both upper extremities WFL, knee extension lacks 10 degrees and flexion is limited to 75 degrees

Strength: Both upper extremities WFL

Pain: Right knee pain reported as 4/10 at rest and 7/10 when standing

Functional mobility and transfers: Client needs minimal assistance sit ↔ stand and contact guard assistance to ambulate using a walker.

Activity tolerance: Activity tolerance for standing is limited to approximately 5 minutes due to post-surgical knee pain and stiffness.

BADL: Requires minimal assistance for lower body bathing and moderate assistance to place underwear and pants over right foot and to don right sock and shoe.

In collaboration with the OT, which of the following equipment, adaptive devices, or interventions are likely appropriate for an OTA to use with Harvey at this time to address his deficits? Assume that interventions would include not only the provision of a particular piece of equipment or DME, but actual instruction and practice in its use. Mark Y (yes) or N (no).

1. _____ Raised toilet seat

2. _____ Tub seat/bench

3. _____ Pillow under right knee when lying in bed

4. _____ Buttonhook

5. _____ Long-handled shoehorn

6. _____ Commode

7. _____ Hot pack to right knee

8. _____ Elastic shoelaces

9. _____ Sock aid

10. _____ Reacher

11. _____ Beanbag toss activity while seated on mat

12. _____ Ambulation using parallel bars

13. _____ Squatting exercises to increase knee ROM

14. _____ Using ambulation device while obtaining items from refrigerator

15. _____ Standing to make a sandwich

Morreale, M. J. (2015). *Developing clinical competence: A workbook for the OTA.* Thorofare, NJ: SLACK Incorporated.

Worksheet 5-5 (continued)

Total Knee Replacement Interventions

16. _____ Power wheelchair mobility training

17. _____ Pegboard activity

18. _____ Cone stacking activity with wrist weights

19. _____ Standing at bathroom sink to shave with electric razor

20. _____ Ambulating up and down the hallway

Worksheet 5-6

Activities as Interventions—Using a Menu

Occupational therapy practitioners work with clients who have brain injuries, intellectual disabilities, mental health conditions, or problems with social interaction. It is beneficial to incorporate activities and occupations during therapy sessions as an effective means to increase the client's occupational performance. For this exercise, determine 10 ways in which a **menu** can be used in occupational therapy to improve specific mental functions, process skills, or social interaction skills needed for various occupations, either by role-playing (using a take-out menu or the menu on a restaurant website) or going to the on-site cafeteria or another eating establishment in the community. List the occupation category, client factor/performance skill being addressed, along with the specific intervention task and methods of implementation. Two examples are provided.

Occupation	Client Factor/Performance Skill to Be Addressed	Specific Intervention Activity	Method (i.e., Role-Play, Menu Choices, Educate Client)
IADL—Financial management	Improve calculation skills	Select an appetizer, entrée, and dessert that total less than $20.00 before tax and tip	Choose items from menu Teach math skills
IADL—Health management	Demonstrate healthy food choices Improve problem solving	Choose an entrée and side dish that are not deep fried	Choose items from menu Educate client regarding healthy versus unhealthy foods and emotional eating (i.e., comfort foods)

Morreale, M. J. (2015). *Developing clinical competence: A workbook for the OTA.* Thorofare, NJ: SLACK Incorporated.

Learning Activity 5-2: Activities as Interventions— Using a Newspaper

Occupational therapy practitioners work with clients who have brain injuries, intellectual disabilities, mental health conditions, or problems with social interaction. It is beneficial to incorporate activities and occupations during therapy sessions as an effective means to increase the client's occupational performance. For this exercise, determine 10 ways in which a **newspaper** can be used in occupational therapy to improve specific mental functions or process skills needed for various occupations. For each of your tasks, determine how it might change the task demands if you were to use a "real" newspaper instead of a Web-based newspaper. List the occupation category, client factor/performance skill being addressed, along with the specific intervention activity. Two examples are provided.

Occupation	Client Factor/ Performance Skill to Be Addressed	Specific Intervention Activity	A "Real" Newspaper Versus a Web-Based Newspaper
Leisure participation	Improve scanning/visual field awareness	Scan page to find TV schedule for a specific time of day	A "real" newspaper opened up provides a much larger area for scanning
IADL—Community mobility	Improve problem solving and topographical orientation	Read a restaurant review and then figure out directions to get there	A web-based newspaper may have a link for directions to the restaurant

© SLACK Incorporated, 2015.

Morreale, M. J. (2015). *Developing clinical competence: A workbook for the OTA*. Thorofare, NJ: SLACK Incorporated.

Learning Activity 5-3: Activities as Interventions— Using a Food Circular

Occupational therapy practitioners work with clients who have brain injuries, intellectual disabilities, mental health conditions, or problems with social interaction. It is beneficial to incorporate activities and occupations during therapy sessions as an effective means to increase the client's occupational performance. For this exercise, determine 10 ways in which a **food sale circular** can be used in occupational therapy to improve specific mental functions, process skills, or social interaction skills needed for occupational performance. List the occupation category, client factor/performance skill being addressed, along with the specific intervention activity. Two examples are provided.

Occupation	Client Factor/Performance Skill to be Addressed	Specific Intervention Activity
IADL—Shopping and financial management	Improve categorization skills	Match a stack of coupons to items that are listed in the food circular
IADL—Shopping Social participation	Improve assertiveness skills	Request a rain check for an advertised sale item that is not in stock

Morreale, M. J. (2015). *Developing clinical competence: A workbook for the OTA.* Thorofare, NJ: SLACK Incorporated.

Worksheet 5-7

Improving Basic and Instrumental Activities of Daily Living Occupations—More Practice

1. A client diagnosed with dysphagia has dietary restrictions that allow only puréed foods and liquids with a nectar consistency. The client also exhibits fair upper extremity muscle strength. Which of the following primary methods is appropriate for the OTA to implement when teaching this client feeding skills?

   A. Position client sitting in a chair and using a straw to sip plain apple juice

   B. Position client sitting in a chair and using a large-handled spoon to eat cream of tomato soup

   C. Position client sitting in a chair and using a built-up spoon to eat scrambled eggs

   D. Position client sitting in a chair and using a chin tuck and a two-handled cup when sipping plain milk

2. An OTA is working in a rehabilitation hospital with a 72-year-old client who sustained a right CVA 2 weeks ago. The client is beginning to demonstrate some limited motor return for left scapula and glenohumeral motions but exhibits subluxation at the glenohumeral joint. The client also requires moderate assistance to transfer to the bed, wheelchair, and toilet. Which of the following devices is most appropriate for the OTA use at this time to address the client's upper extremity deficits?

   A. Airplane splint

   B. Arm trough

   C. Pulleys

   D. Therapy putty

3. An OTA is working with a 52-year-old client who exhibits left upper and lower extremity hemiplegia. The client requires assistance for self-care tasks and is presently unable to perform functional ambulation independently. Which of the following devices is probably the least useful for the OTA to recommend at this time?

   A. Plate guard

   B. Hand-held shower head

   C. Rolling walker

   D. Buttonhook

4. An OTA is working with a client who has a diagnosis of right macular degeneration. In order to help compensate for deficits associated with this condition, the OTA should recommend which of the following devices?

   A. Hearing aid

   B. Magnifying glass

   C. Sock assist

   D. Forearm-based thumb spica splint

5. An OTA is working with an older adult who lives alone. The client is diagnosed with a vestibular problem that is creating safety concerns. In order to help compensate for deficits associated with this condition, which of the following devices is most useful for the OTA to recommend?

   A. Use a tub seat when bathing

   B. Install a fire alarm that uses strobe lights

   C. Use backless rubber-soled slippers when performing functional ambulation at home

   D. Pull up from walker when transferring sit to stand

Worksheet 5-7 (continued)

Improving Basic and Instrumental Activities of Daily Living Occupations—More Practice

6. An OTA is working with an older adult who lives alone and is diagnosed with bilateral presbycusis. In order to help compensate for deficits associated with this condition, which of the following devices is most useful for the OTA to recommend?

    A. Reacher

    B. Elevated toilet seat

    C. Sock assist

    D. Telephone amplifier

7. An OTA is working with a male client who has severe COPD and sustained a Colle's fracture of his dominant right arm. The client's cast was removed last week and he has difficulty grasping and manipulating objects. Which of the following interventions is most appropriate for the OTA to implement at this time to improve the client's hand function?

    A. Exercising with pulleys

    B. Fluidotherapy

    C. Buttoning a shirt

    D. Sanding and staining a wood birdhouse

8. An OTA's primary role in hospice care is which of the following?

    A. Teach bed mobility and transfers

    B. Fabricate splints and teach proper positioning

    C. Implement interventions to support occupational engagement

    D. Improve upper body strength

9. A 32-year-old client with a hand amputation has an upper limb prosthesis classified as a passive terminal device. During prosthetic training, which of the following is most appropriate for the OTA to have the client do with the prosthetic hand?

    A. Perform sensory activities to help distinguish hot and cold water

    B. Perform sensory activities to help distinguish sharp from dull objects

    C. Attempt to use it as a gross assist

    D. Test the battery before attempting a functional task

10. A 45-year-old client with an upper extremity amputation is learning how to use his myoelectric prosthesis. During prosthetic training, which of the following is most appropriate for the OTA to have the client do with the prosthetic hand?

    A. Attempt to pick up a foam cup

    B. Perform sensory activities to help distinguish hot and cold

    C. Practice isolated finger motion for buttoning a shirt

    D. Perform finger to palm translation using coins

Worksheet 5-8

Fracture Interventions

Abe, a 64-year-old male, sustained a scaphoid fracture in his dominant right upper extremity secondary to a motor vehicle accident. The cast was removed 2 days ago and Abe was referred to outpatient occupational therapy. The prescription states, *"OT for RUE P/AROM, PAMs PRN, and ADL/IADL retraining; 3 times weekly for 4 weeks."*

Here is some information taken from Abe's initial evaluation report.

Medical history: Parkinson's disease, degenerative joint disease left hip, and history of kidney stones

Prior level of function: Lives with wife in a garden apartment. Retired 4 years ago from his job teaching high school science. Client was independent in BADL and IADL except for driving, which he stopped doing 1 year ago due to Parkinson's effects.

Edema: None noted in right upper extremity

Pain: Right wrist reported as 6/10

Sensation: Intact

Upper extremity ROM:

- Bilateral resting tremors noted
- Left upper extremity: WNL
- Right upper extremity: Shoulder and elbow WNL
- Forearm pronation 0/76, supination 0/54
- Wrist flexion 0/42, extension 0/32, ulnar deviation 0/14, radial deviation 0/8
- Client presents with moderate stiffness in right hand, inability to flex fingers to touch palm, opposition only to index finger

Functional mobility and transfers: Client able to perform functional ambulation and transfers independently with slightly increased time. Reports pain in left hip when standing (5/10).

BADL/IADL: Since his injury, client reports difficulty performing activities requiring grip or fine-motor skills, such as managing clothing fastenings, shaving, brushing teeth, eating, writing, performing home maintenance.

The intervention plan for Abe includes goals to increase right wrist and hand ROM/strength to enable modified independence in BADL. In collaboration with the OT, which of the following equipment, adaptive devices, or adapted techniques might be appropriate for an OTA to use with Abe during therapy the first 2 weeks to address his primary deficits? Assume that interventions would include not only the provision of a particular piece of equipment or DME, but actual instruction and practice in its use. Mark Y (yes) or N (no).

1. _____ Built-up pen

2. _____ Pegboard

3. _____ Built-up utensils

4. _____ Arm push-ups while sitting on mat

5. _____ Universal cuff

6. _____ Paraffin to right hand

7. _____ Sock aid

8. _____ Retrograde massage

9. _____ Vigorous stretching to wrist

Worksheet 5-8 (continued)
Fracture Interventions

10. _____ Elastic shoelaces

11. _____ MP extension resting splint

12. _____ Wash mitt

13. _____ Practice transfers using a raised toilet seat

14. _____ Sensory retraining

15. _____ Towel scrunching with fingers

16. _____ Shoes with Velcro closures

17. _____ Hot pack to wrist

18. _____ Hot pack to left hip

19. _____ Pulleys

20. _____ Walker

Worksheet 5-9

Chronic Obstructive Pulmonary Disease Interventions

Frank is a 72-year-old male residing with his wife, who has dementia, in an assisted living facility. He recently experienced an exacerbation of COPD, was admitted to an acute care hospital for 3 days, and then transferred to a rehabilitation hospital where he is presently. Frank worked as a painter but retired at age 58 due to respiratory ailments. In addition to the medications needed to address his respiratory problems, Frank has been taking Coumadin (warfarin) since being diagnosed with atrial fibrillation 2 years ago. Prior to this recent hospitalization, Frank drove a car, could manage BADL with increased time, and used a rollator walker when not in his room. Frank is currently on portable oxygen. He needs minimal assistance to perform transfers, moderate assistance to complete lower body bathing and dressing, and cannot stand for more than 2 minutes without shortness of breath. Upper extremity ROM is WNL. In collaboration with the OT, which of the following equipment, adaptive devices, or interventions are likely appropriate for an OTA to use with Frank to improve performance skills and client factors and enable return to his residence? Assume that interventions would include not only the provision of a particular piece of equipment or DME, but actual instruction and practice in its use. Mark Y (yes) or N (no).

1. _____ Raised toilet seat

2. _____ One-arm-drive wheelchair

3. _____ Instruction in joint protection

4. _____ Buttonhook

5. _____ Sanding and painting wood

6. _____ Commode

7. _____ Hot pack to shoulders

8. _____ Safety razor

9. _____ Exercise bands

10. _____ Reacher

11. _____ Ergonomics for yard work

12. _____ Standing while playing a game

13. _____ Energy conservation for doing laundry

14. _____ Using ambulation device while getting clothes from dresser

15. _____ Standing to cook at stove

16. _____ Pursed lip breathing

17. _____ Long-handled shoehorn

18. _____ Sawing and staining wood to make a picture frame

19. _____ Teaching stair climbing

20. _____ Shampoo and soap dispenser in shower

Morreale, M. J. (2015). *Developing clinical competence: A workbook for the OTA*. Thorofare, NJ: SLACK Incorporated.

Worksheet 5-10

Meal Preparation Adaptations

Carmen is a 65-year-old homemaker who sustained a left CVA 2 weeks ago. She lives with her husband in a private home and was fully independent in all ADL prior to this illness. At the present time, Carmen's cognition appears to be intact, but she exhibits Broca's aphasia and right hemiparesis. Her dominant right upper extremity is beginning to exhibit minimal motor return but is essentially nonfunctional except for some gross stabilization of objects. The client also demonstrates modified independence for functional ambulation using a hemi-walker. However, Carmen is unsafe when bending to reach for objects in lower kitchen cabinets. Her activity tolerance for standing is approximately 4 minutes. In each of the boxes below, list several suggestions indicating how the following breakfast tasks can be adapted to help enable safe and independent performance.

Adaptive Equipment and Compensatory Methods	Scrambled Eggs	Bacon	Fresh Fruit Salad (apple, grapes, pear, strawberries)	Pancakes
Required tools/ equipment (list adaptive equipment or compensatory methods)	*Example: Use a nonstick pan for easier clean up*			
Required supplies (food items)	*Example: Use a cooking spray to grease pan*			
Required actions and timing	*Example: Sit, rather than stand, at stove*			

Morreale, M. J. (2015). *Developing clinical competence: A workbook for the OTA.* Thorofare, NJ: SLACK Incorporated.

Learning Activity 5-4: School Occupations

For each of the following student weaknesses in performance skills or client factors, list three educationally related activities that may be impacted by those weaknesses in a school setting. Examples are provided for each category.

Area of Weakness	Educationally Related Activity That May Be Impacted in a School Setting
Tactile sensory processing	1. Art class project using glue 2. 3. 4.
Organizational skills	1. Writing down all homework assignments and developing a timeline for completion 2. 3. 4.
Proprioception	1. Applying appropriate amount of pressure to avoid breakage of pencil or crayon when writing or coloring 2. 3. 4.
Time management	1. Getting to next class in allotted time frame 2. 3. 4.
Fine-motor skills	1. Managing fastenings on clothing when changing for gym class 2. 3. 4.
Grip strength	1. Carrying lunch box 2. 3. 4.

Area of Weakness	Educationally Related Activity That May Be Impacted in a School Setting
Standing balance/ tolerance	*1. Standing in line to purchase lunch in cafeteria* 2. 3. 4.
Shoulder ROM	*1. Hanging clothing in locker* 2. 3. 4.
Upper extremity strength	*1. Carrying books* 2. 3. 4.
Eye-hand coordination	*1. Opening combination lock on locker* 2. 3. 4.
Crossing midline	*1. Turning pages in a large book* 2. 3. 4.
Spatial relations	*1. Buckling school bus seat belt* 2. 3. 4.

Morreale, M. J. (2015). *Developing clinical competence: A workbook for the OTA*. Thorofare, NJ: SLACK Incorporated.

Area of Weakness	Educationally Related Activity That May Be Impacted in a School Setting
Bilateral integration	1. Washing hands after toileting 2. 3. 4.
Visual-motor	1. Copying notes from the blackboard 2. 3. 4.
Categorization	1. Sorting school papers according to subject 2. 3. 4.
Calculation skills	1. Calculating cost of two items at school bake sale and the change back from $1.00 2. 3. 4.
Emotional regulation	1. When walking in a line going to the cafeteria or school bus, remaining calm when accidentally getting bumped by a classmate 2. 3. 4.

Morreale, M. J. (2015). *Developing clinical competence: A workbook for the OTA*. Thorofare, NJ: SLACK Incorporated.

Worksheet 5-11

Supported Employment

Joe is a 20-year-old male with Down syndrome. He attends a supported employment program with the goal for him to work in a grocery store packing groceries. Joe does not have any physical limitations that would hinder his job performance. However, he does exhibit difficulty with time management and transitioning between activities. Joe needs to learn how to perform his job functions correctly, including interacting appropriately with customers. Consider the activity demands for a grocery packing job. Use a professional format to list six goals for Joe that relate to his employment and reflect the categories listed below.

Example: Joe will be able to complete grocery packing for three customers without asking when he can take a break, within 2 months.

1. Time management

2. Activity transition

3. Social interaction

4. Packing groceries (specific aspect)

5. Packing groceries (specific aspect)

6. Packing groceries (specific aspect)

Morreale, M. J. (2015). *Developing clinical competence: A workbook for the OTA.* Thorofare, NJ: SLACK Incorporated.

Answers to Worksheets

The worksheets in this chapter delineate only select interventions that may not be appropriate for all clients with that condition. A client situation may also warrant other types of interventions or devices that are not included here.

Worksheet 5-1: Teaching-Learning Process (Total Hip Replacement)

Each intervention session will vary in terms of specific tasks performed and the order implemented depending on the client's medical status, level of function, doctor's orders, time frames, client tolerance, etc., but here are some suggestions:

1. Where will the session take place? *Client's hospital room*

2. What is the anticipated length of session? *15 to 45 minutes as per client's tolerance*

3. What equipment/supplies will the OTA need to bring to the session?

    A. *Documentation materials (i.e., laptop/hand-held device, paper, pen, documentation forms)*

    B. *Adaptive equipment: sock aid, reacher, dressing stick, long-handled shoehorn, elastic laces*

    C. *Gloves/personal protective equipment for potential contact with blood or body fluids*

    D. *Written client education materials*

    E. *Ensure walker is in room*

    F. *Hospital scrubs for dressing practice if client does not have street clothes in room*

    G. *As needed, stethoscope or other equipment to assess vital signs*

4. What are several things the OTA should do prior to entering the client's room?

    A. *Collaborate with OT and review the occupational therapy evaluation report and intervention plan*

    B. *Establish OTA's schedule and coordinate time frames with physical therapy/other disciplines as needed*

    C. *Check client's chart for changes in medical status and new orders and review nursing, physical therapy documentation, and other sections as indicated*

    D. *Obtain any further knowledge needed regarding this diagnosis or client's condition*

    E. *Carefully consider any precautions/contraindications and safety concerns for this client, as well as pertinent infection control issues*

    F. *Double check that this is the correct room and correct patient (i.e., check wrist band, verbally ask client)*

5. List the general steps of how the session should be implemented:

    A. *Perform hand hygiene and use personal protective equipment as indicated*

    B. *Introduce OTA and explain purpose of session (refer back to Chapter 1)*

    C. *Note any devices hooked up to client requiring caution during treatment such as a catheter, monitor, or IV*

    D. *Take vital signs if part of protocol or as indicated during session*

    E. *Review general total hip precautions and determine client understanding and carryover*

    F. *Ensure bed brakes are locked and adjust bed rail as needed. Explain transfer procedure then transfer client safely to a sitting position (on edge of bed or into a chair depending on client's status and intervention plan) adhering to total hip precautions and using walker and safe client footwear if performing stand-pivot transfer.*

    G. *Explain/demonstrate use of adaptive devices for lower body dressing, one at a time*

    H. *Following each explanation/demonstration, have client practice use of adaptive equipment to don lower body clothing/scrubs while adhering to precautions and providing assistance as needed. Incorporate use of walker and provide contact guard/physical assist when client stands to pull up clothing.*

    I. *Provide opportunities for problem solving and client feedback*

    J. *Determine if client needs to practice using any of the devices a second time this session (or future sessions), or if clothing needs to removed and hospital gown put back on*

    K. *Client may also don upper body clothing if indicated*

    L. *Transfer client back to bed or determine if client should remain sitting in chair*

    M. *Make sure equipment is properly placed and client is comfortable and safe and can reach the call button*

N. *Dispose of any personal protective equipment or used linens properly*

O. *Wash hands*

P. *Document according to facility time frame*

Changes in the teaching-learning process for a 90-year-old client would depend on various factors, such as the client's prior level of function. Depending on the expected discharge plan, lower body dressing may or may not be a priority for this client (i.e., lived alone independently versus resided in a nursing home). If the client were 90 years old with age-related hearing loss or visual impairment, you might have to ensure that hearing aids are in place or use large-print educational materials. Processing may be slower, so the client may need greater task breakdown or additional opportunities to practice new skills. In addition, the client may require more rest breaks.

Worksheet 5-2: Cerebrovascular Accident Interventions

Suggested resources: Gillen, 2011; Logigian, 2005; Morawski & Padilla, 2012

1. Y. Rocker knife

2. Y. Nonslip matting

3. N. Built-up utensils
Client is unable to use flaccid right hand and should not need built-up utensils for his unaffected left hand.

4. Y. Plate guard

5. N. Walker
This requires two hands, and client cannot grip walker with a flaccid hand. Physical therapy will determine when a hemi-walker is appropriate for client to use.

6. N. Power wheelchair
Client should be able to operate a manual wheelchair using his left arm and leg or a one-arm-drive wheelchair.

7. Y. Electric razor

8. N. Sock aid
Client cannot use right hand, so it would be difficult to use this device one-handed. It would probably be better to teach one-handed compensatory techniques.

9. N. Therapy putty
Cannot use with flaccid right hand.

10. N. Exercise bands
Cannot use with flaccid right upper extremity.

11. N. Pulleys
Using pulleys for PROM to a flaccid right upper extremity may overstretch joints/cause harm to the shoulder.

12. N. Vest restraint
A vest restraint is not appropriate. If Marvin is demonstrating poor posture in chair, other less restrictive alternatives should be tried, such as client education, verbal reminders, lateral cushions/supports, a seatbelt that client can manage, etc.

13. Y. Wheelchair arm support

14. Y. Soap-on-a-rope

15. Y. Wash mitt

16. Y. Soap/shampoo dispenser

17. Y. Long-handled sponge

18. Y. Tub seat/bench

19. N. Hot pack to right shoulder
Not indicated for a flaccid extremity with no pain or PROM deficits. Also, cardiovascular status may not be stable.

20. N. Paraffin to right hand
Not indicated for a flaccid extremity with no pain or PROM deficits. Also, cardiovascular status may not be stable.

21. N. Constraint-induced movement therapy
Client does not have the requisite motor skills in his involved arm for this intervention as the arm is flaccid. Constraining the strong arm would not allow the client to perform any functional tasks at this time.

22. Y. Teach self-ROM

23. N. Lapboard
    This could be considered a restraint if the client is not able to remove it himself. Other alternatives should be tried first, such as a side-arm support.

24. N. Large pegboard
    Client's involved arm is flaccid, and this task would not be useful for the uninvolved arm. If the client had perceptual deficits it could possibly be used with the unaffected arm to work on specific perceptual skills, although a functional task would be more appropriate.

25. N. Nine-Hole Peg Test
    Client does not have any motor function in his involved dominant right upper extremity, so this test would not be a useful measure at this time.

Worksheet 5-3: Total Hip Replacement Interventions

Suggested resources: Coppard, Higgins, Harvey, & Padilla, 2012; Gower & Bowker, 2005; Maher & Bear-Lehman, 2008

1. Y. Raised toilet seat

2. N. Adduction cushion
   Client needs an abduction cushion.

3. N. Built-up utensils

4. Y. Commode

5. N. Crossing legs to tie shoes
   Unable to adduct hip due to surgical precautions.

6. Y. Walker
   Generally, the PT would determine if this device is appropriate for gait training at this time. However, occupational therapy can support functional mobility and safety for occupational performance.

7. N. Power wheelchair
   A manual wheelchair is typically more appropriate following hip replacement surgery.

8. Y. Long-handled shoehorn

9. Y. Sock aid

10. N. Hot pack to left hip
    A hot pack is not indicated for acute post-surgical conditions, but a cold pack might be appropriate for pain and swelling. State regulation and facility policy delineate the disciplines that may apply particular physical agents.

11. N. Paraffin to left hand
    Not indicated for client's condition as no ROM deficits are noted.

12. N. Teach stair climbing with crutches
    Teaching stair climbing is typically the role of the PT, although occupational therapy can support function. Crutches are not an appropriate mobility device for this client due to her age and functional level.

13. N. Wheelchair arm support
    Client does not have unilateral neglect or ROM deficits.

14. Y. Exercise bands
    Increasing upper body strength may be beneficial for walker use.

15. N. Quad cane
    Cannot use with non-weight-bearing status.

16. Y. Elastic shoelaces

17. N. Wedge cushion for wheelchair
    This would provide excessive hip flexion. However, an elevated seat cushion would be appropriate.

18. Y. Reacher

19. Y. Long-handled sponge

20. Y. Tub seat/bench

21. Y. Leg lifter
Useful to help lift involved lower limb when transferring to a tub bench or bed.

22. N. Constraint-induced movement therapy
This technique is useful for clients with neurological conditions, such as stroke, to improve upper limb function (Gillen, 2011). Client does not have neurological impairment and has good voluntary motion in both upper extremities.

23. N. Sliding board
Instruction in stand-pivot transfers is a more appropriate method for this client and condition.

24. N. Buttonhook
Client has full AROM in both upper extremities and no coordination deficits are noted.

25. N. Hospital bed for home
Client has potential for good bed mobility and does not have another condition that would warrant use of a hospital bed, such as respiratory problems.

Worksheet 5-4: Improving Basic and Instrumental Activities of Daily Living Occupations

1. A. Minor & Minor, 2006.

2. B. The client should be able to transfer independently onto the commode using a sliding board. A raised toilet seat is not useful, as the client cannot enter the bathroom. Using a platform walker is not feasible. A power mobility scooter may not fit through the door or, most likely, will not be able to get close enough to the toilet for a sliding board transfer.

3. C. The client's knees should be apart to provide a wider base of support. A transfer belt could be placed around the client's waist, but not the OTA's. A walker is unstable as a device to push up from, so this would be unsafe. The client needs to lean forward ("nose over toes") to facilitate rising from chair.

4. C. An electric razor is safer than a safety razor that has sharp blades. As the client has unilateral neglect and impulsivity, he needs to focus all his attention on the task at hand to best perform shaving. Standing would be more distracting in this case, as the client would have to work to maintain his balance. However, realize there are instances when an occupational therapy practitioner would work on balance (or other client factors) and ADL performance simultaneously, depending on the desired outcome for that session.

5. B. Clients should be as upright as possible when feeding. Neck hyperextension would hinder swallowing and could be unsafe (Morawski, Davis, & Padilla, 2012). Specialized swallowing techniques or alternate neck positions may be needed for some clients. If weakness is only evident in the hand intrinsic muscles, the client should be able to manage self-feeding with a universal cuff or adapted utensils.

6. A. The best strategy would be to teach an easier method, which in this case is over-the-head. While demonstration and written instructions could help, they are not the best option. A larger coat would still require the same sequence of motor planning.

7. D. Using a flat sheet as a bottom sheet entails less effort than using a fitted sheet. While a tub seat is useful, it is not related to homemaking. It is contraindicated to use open flames (barbecue grill) around oxygen. The client should inhale before exertion and exhale during the exertion.

8. D. Driving is not feasible at this level, whereas the other interventions are appropriate (Fike, Pendleton, & Hewitt, 2005; Spinal Cord Injury Information Pages, 2013).

9. D. The triceps are not innervated at this level, but the client may be able to shift sideways to relieve pressure. Using a buttonhook and razor are feasible, but may require set up and use of a holder or a tenodesis grasp wrist-driven hinge orthosis (Fike et al., 2005; Spinal Cord Injury Information Pages, 2013).

10. B. The client is able to use a manual wheelchair at this level. The client should be able to perform many functional tasks, such as light meal preparation and bathing. As the triceps are innervated at this level, the client should be instructed in wheelchair push-ups to help relieve pressure while sitting (Fike et al., 2005; Spinal Cord Injury Information Pages, 2013).

Worksheet 5-5: Total Knee Replacement Interventions

Suggested resources: Coppard et al., 2012

1. Y. Raised toilet seat
Could be useful.

2. Y. Tub seat/bench

3. N. Pillow under right knee when lying in bed
A pillow under the affected knee can contribute to a knee flexion contracture, which is undesirable.

4. N. Buttonhook
There are no upper extremity deficits noted.

5. Y. Long-handled shoehorn

6. Y. Commode

7. N. Hot pack to right knee
A hot pack is not indicated for acute post-surgical conditions, but a cold pack might be appropriate for pain and swelling. State regulation and facility policy delineate the disciplines that may apply particular physical agents.

8. Y. Elastic shoelaces

9. Y. Sock aid
May not need though.

10. Y. Reacher

11. N. Beanbag toss activity while seated on mat
Sitting balance is not a problem.

12. N. Ambulation using parallel bars
This is typically a physical therapy intervention.

13. N. Squatting exercises to increase knee ROM
This is typically a physical therapy intervention; knee may be unstable postoperatively.

14. Y. Using ambulation device while obtaining items from refrigerator
Realize that while activity tolerance for standing is an important goal for this client and condition, this activity may increase pain. The occupational therapy practitioner must decide if the client would benefit more from a compensatory method, such as using a wheelchair, or determine if the client needs to work through the pain, depending on physician orders and the client's particular situation.

15. Y. Standing to make a sandwich
Realize that while activity tolerance for standing is an important goal for this client and condition, this activity may increase pain. The occupational therapy practitioner must decide if the client would benefit more from a compensatory method, such as sitting on a chair at the kitchen counter, or determine if the client needs to work through the pain, depending on physician orders and the client's particular situation.

16. N. Power wheelchair mobility training
Power wheelchair is not needed.

17. N. Pegboard activity
No fine-motor deficits indicated.

18. N. Cone stacking activity with wrist weights
Could possibly use to increase endurance, but strength is already WFL and client has other ADL priorities. Can use while standing to work on improving standing tolerance.

19. Y. Standing at bathroom sink to shave with electric razor
Realize that while activity tolerance for standing is an important goal for this client and condition, this activity may increase pain. The occupational therapy practitioner must decide if the client would benefit more from a compensatory method, such as sitting in a chair at the sink, or determine if the client needs to work through the pain, depending on physician orders and the client's particular situation.

20. N. Ambulating up and down the hallway
Ambulation training is typically a physical therapy intervention, although occupational therapy can support functional mobility for occupations, such as safe navigation in the kitchen during meal preparation tasks.

Worksheet 5-6: Activities as Interventions—Using a Menu

Here are some suggestions although you may come up with others. While the methods listed next include the activity of role-playing, an occupational therapy practitioner should create opportunities to have clients perform real occupations, such as actually going to a restaurant.

Occupation	Client Factor/Performance Skill to Be Addressed	Specific Intervention Activity	Method (i.e., Role-Play, Menu Choices, Educate Client)
IADL—Financial management	Improve calculation skills	Select an appetizer, entrée, and dessert that total less than $20.00 before tax and tip	Choose items from menu Teach math skills
IADL—Health management	Demonstrate healthy food choices Improve problem solving Improve coping skills	Choose an entrée and side dish that are not deep fried	Choose items from menu Educate client regarding healthy versus unhealthy foods and emotional eating (i.e., comfort foods)
IADL—Health management	Demonstrate healthy drinking choices Improve coping skills	Choose a beverage that does not contain alcohol, or choose a beverage that will or will not add calories, depending on the client's dietary needs	Choose items from menu Educate client regarding healthy versus unhealthy beverage choices and emotional eating Role-play and suggest coping strategies
IADL—Health management	Improve problem solving Improve safety awareness	Determine items that may contain allergens such as nuts, dairy products, or gluten	Choose items from menu Educate client regarding hidden ingredients
Leisure participation Social participation	Improve decision-making skills	Within a 5-minute period, choose a beverage, entrée, and dessert without changing mind, or choose a restaurant for the group to go to	Role-play and provide feedback
Leisure participation Social participation	Improve assertiveness skills	Ask the server for something not already on the table, such as a glass of water, extra napkins, or a condiment	Role-play and provide feedback
IADL—Health management	Demonstrate healthy eating habits Improve assertiveness skills	Ask server how an item is prepared, or ask for item to be specially prepared without butter, salt, etc.	Role-play and provide feedback
BADL—Feeding Social participation	Improve problem solving	Choose items that one can manage to eat without need for help or set-up	Choose items from menu (i.e., finger foods or fish fillet that does not need to be cut) Educate regarding compensatory strategies
IADL—Health management	Demonstrate healthy eating habits	Choose an appetizer, entrée, and beverage that total less or more than a specified amount of calories or sodium	Choose items from menu Educate client regarding healthy versus unhealthy foods and emotional response to food

Occupation	Client Factor/Performance Skill to Be Addressed	Specific Intervention Activity	Method (i.e., Role-Play, Menu Choices, Educate Client)
IADL—Financial management	Improve calculation skills	Calculate tax and tip on specified items	Choose items from menu Teach math skills
IADL—Financial management	Improve calculation skills	Determine change back from a $50.00 bill after selecting several items	Choose items from menu Teach math skills
IADL—Financial management	Improve money management	Pay using exact change or perform credit card transaction properly	Role-play
Social participation	Improve interpersonal skills	Choose an appetizer or dessert that can be shared with the group	Choose items from menu Role-play and provide feedback

Worksheet 5-7: Improving Basic and Instrumental Activities of Daily Living Occupations—More Practice

1. B. Plain apple juice and milk are thin liquids that the client is not allowed to have. If thickeners were added to create a nectar consistency, they might be acceptable. Scrambled eggs are soft, but semi-solid, and not considered to be puréed. It is essential to know what is acceptable or not acceptable for each client to eat. Clients may have dairy restrictions, food allergies, cultural considerations, or require special diets due to other medical concerns (i.e., a low-sodium or low-sugar diet).

2. B. As the client must use a wheelchair, an arm trough may be helpful to support and protect the involved arm. An airplane splint is a shoulder immobilization splint, which is not indicated for this condition. Pulleys may cause further damage to the shoulder if the arm is overstretched, and the client also does not have the requisite grasp to manage this device or to use therapy putty with the left hand.

3. C. The client does not have the requisite function of the involved arm to hold onto a rolling walker. The other devices may be used to teach the client compensatory techniques for ADL.

4. B. Macular degeneration is an eye disease. Only one of the choices relates to vision.

5. A. Vestibular problems may create vertigo or problems with balance. It is probably best that the client be seated while bathing. When going from sit to stand, the client should push up from the seated surface rather than pull up from a walker, which would be unsafe. Slippers without a back do not provide proper stability and may cause the foot to slide, possibly contributing to a fall. While the client should have a fire alarm in the home, strobe lights are not needed.

6. D. Presbycusis is an age-related hearing loss. The only choice that relates to hearing is a telephone amplifier.

7. C. Due to the client's diagnosis of COPD, the OTA should avoid activities that may create dust (such as Fluidotherapy and sanding) or fumes (staining wood). While use of pulleys may involve grasp, this device is not the best choice to facilitate hand function. A functional fine-motor task, such as buttoning a shirt, is a better choice.

8. C. While A, B, and D are possible interventions that an occupational therapy practitioner might provide to clients receiving hospice care, these interventions are not needed for every client. An occupational therapy practitioner considers each client individually to determine appropriate interventions to help support the client's desired or needed occupational roles and quality of life (AOTA, 2011).

9. C. An upper limb prosthesis classified as a passive terminal device does not have a battery. It is primarily used for cosmesis but can possibly be used as a gross assist (Papdapoulos & Deverix, 2013).

10. A. A myoelectric prosthesis can perform grasp but does not have sensory function, isolated motion of digits, or the ability to perform in-hand manipulation. Training includes working on ability to pick up various kinds of objects without damaging the objects (Papdapoulos & Deverix, 2013).

Worksheet 5-8: Fracture Interventions

Suggested resources: Coppard et al., 2012

1. Y. Built-up pen
2. Y. Pegboard
    However, it is better to perform functional activities such as buttoning a shirt.
3. Y. Built-up utensils
4. N. Arm push-ups while sitting on mat
    Contraindicated at this time. May cause excessive pressure on healing fracture.
5. Y. Universal cuff
6. N. Paraffin to right hand
    Tremors would create a safety concern for splashing paraffin or touching sides of unit.
7. N. Sock aid
    Client does not have the necessary motor function in hand and tremors also create more difficulty.
8. N. Retrograde massage
    No edema present.
9. N. Vigorous stretching to wrist
    Fracture may not yet be stable enough for vigorous stretching.
10. Y. Elastic shoelaces
11. N. MP extension resting splint
    Except for certain protocols (i.e., extensor tendon repair, MP joint replacement surgery, etc.), the hand generally should not be splinted in MP extension as this is not a functional position.
12. Y. Wash mitt
13. N. Practice transfers using a raised toilet seat
    Client is already independent in transfers, although the OTA may recommend this for the future.
14. N. Sensory retraining
    Sensation is intact
15. Y. Towel scrunching with fingers
16. Y. Shoes with Velcro closures
17. Y. Hot pack to wrist
18. N. Hot pack to left hip
    Client was referred for an upper extremity diagnosis. A referral to physical therapy may be warranted to address the client's hip pain.
19. N. Pulleys
    Client's limited grip creates difficulty for holding the handle. Also, pulleys do not really address client's ROM deficits in hand and wrist.
20. N. Walker
    Client is independent in ambulation. However, a referral to physical therapy may be warranted to determine if an ambulation device is appropriate for this client to minimize hip pain.

Worksheet 5-9: Chronic Obstructive Pulmonary Disease Interventions

Resources: Peralta, Powell, & Plutschack, 2012

1. Y. Raised toilet seat
2. N. One-arm-drive wheelchair
    Client has use of both arms and legs so does not require this particular type of wheelchair.
3. N. Instruction in joint protection
    Client does not have joint problems. Instruction on energy conservation would be more useful.
4. N. Buttonhook
    No fine-motor deficits noted.

5. N. Sanding and painting wood
    Creates dust and fumes.

6. Y. Commode

7. N. Hot pack to shoulders
    No shoulder problems are noted, and heat is contraindicated for severe cardiopulmonary conditions.

8. N. Safety razor
    Client is on blood thinners and should use an electric razor.

9. Y. Exercise bands
    May be useful to increase strength and endurance.

10. Y. Reacher

11. N. Ergonomics for yard work
    Resides in assisted living facility.

12. Y. Standing while playing a game
    Depending on the client's medical status and intervention plan, graded standing tasks may be useful to increase endurance.

13. N. Energy conservation for doing laundry
    Resides in assisted living facility so staff may do laundry.

14. Y. Using ambulation device while getting clothes from dresser
    Grading functional mobility tasks may be useful to increase endurance. However, a compensatory method, such as performing the task while seated in a wheelchair, may be needed to enable independent performance of this occupation.

15. N. Standing to cook at stove
    To increase endurance, this could be used as a purposeful activity, but meals are typically provided at an assisted living facility. Depending on the facility, client may be allowed to use a microwave or coffee-maker. However, a compensatory method, such as performing the task while seated, may be needed to enable independent performance of this occupation.

16. Y. Pursed lip breathing

17. Y. Long-handled shoehorn

18. N. Sawing and staining wood to make a picture frame
    Creates dust and fumes, and client is also on blood thinners.

19. N. Teaching stair climbing
    This is typically the role of physical therapy.

20. Y. Shampoo and soap dispenser in shower
    Eliminates reaching for bottles or lifting them.

Worksheet 5-10: Meal Preparation Adaptations

Here are some suggestions for adaptive equipment and compensatory techniques for this client, although you may come up with others. Realize that the dominant hand is unable to perform grasp. Built-up handled objects would not be needed for the nondominant hand.

Adaptive Equipment and Compensatory Methods	Scrambled Eggs	Bacon	Fresh Fruit Salad (Apple, Grapes, Pear, Strawberries)	Pancakes
Required tools/ equipment (list adaptive equipment or compensatory methods)	Nonstick pan for easier clean-up Can use a microwave instead of stove Nonslip matting to secure bowl Use a bowl with a handle to pour	Can use a microwave instead of stove Nonstick pan for easier clean-up	Adapted cutting board with nails Nonslip matting Apple peeling device Can use an egg slicer to slice berries	Depending on method (i.e., frozen pancakes or using a mix), can use a toaster, toaster oven, microwave, electric griddle, or top of stove. If making batter, use nonslip matting to secure bowl If making batter, use a bowl with a handle to pour or use a batter dispenser Nonstick pan for easier clean-up
Required supplies (food items)	Cooking spray to grease pan Liquid eggs in a carton Frozen prepared eggs	Pre-cooked store bought bacon in dairy section Store-bought bacon bits	Pre-cut bags of fruit in frozen food or refrigerated section of supermarket Canned fruit Pre-cut fresh fruit from a grocery store/ salad bar	Pancakes from a recipe versus a boxed mix. Consider number of ingredients needed such as only water versus needing water, oil, and egg Premade store bought batter from a carton Frozen pancakes Cooking spray to grease pan

Adaptive Equipment and Compensatory Methods	Scrambled Eggs	Bacon	Fresh Fruit Salad (Apple, Grapes, Pear, Strawberries)	Pancakes
Required actions and timing	Sit, rather than stand, at stove Teach one-handed technique to break eggs Can use a carton holder with handle when pouring liquid eggs from a carton Keep items in higher shelves of refrigerator and accessible upper cabinets Rolling cart to move and carry items Apron with pockets to move and carry small objects	Use a scissors to open package Sit, rather than stand, to prepare Keep items in higher shelves of refrigerator and accessible upper cabinets Rolling cart to move and carry items Apron with pockets to move and carry small objects	Can use a suction brush attached to sink to wash fruits Sit, rather than stand, to prepare Keep items in higher shelves of refrigerator and accessible upper cabinets Rolling cart to move and carry items Apron with pockets to move and carry small objects	If eggs are needed, teach one-handed technique to break eggs Sit, rather than stand, to prepare Keep items in higher shelves of refrigerator and accessible upper cabinets Rolling cart to move and carry items Can prepare batter ahead of time Teach compensatory method to open box of pancake mix Apron with pockets to move and carry small objects Can use a carton holder with handle when pouring milk or batter from a carton

Worksheet 5-11: Supported Employment

Resources for goal writing: Gateley & Borcherding, 2012; Morreale & Borcherding, 2013

Goals need to specify a time frame, measurable criteria, and delineate a desired client behavior relating to function. Goals should reflect what the client needs to achieve, not what the occupational therapy practitioner will do as interventions. Here are some suggested goals for this client. Realize that different settings or practice areas may use slightly different formats or terminology, as shown in the various examples following. Of course the actual goals and time frames may be different for a real client.

1. Time management
   o By the end of 1 month, Joe will demonstrate ability to pack 10 items in a grocery bag within a 2-minute period.
   o Joe will adhere to the allotted time for breaks with one verbal cue to set and use a timer, within 2 weeks.
2. Activity transition
   o After placing a grocery bag in customer's cart, Joe will continue packing remaining groceries without redirection to task, within 4 weeks.
   o At the end of his allotted break time, client will punch his time card with two verbal cues, within 10 days.
3. Social interaction
   o With one verbal cue, client will ask customers if they prefer paper or plastic bags, 5 out of 5 opportunities, within 2 weeks.
   o Joe will greet customers with a smile and say "hello" 4/5 opportunities, by the end of the month.

4. Packing groceries
   o Within 6 weeks, Joe will demonstrate ability to pack cold items together with minimal verbal cues.
5. Packing groceries
   o Client will demonstrate ability to place cans and heavier items on the bottom of grocery bag with stand-by assist, within 4 weeks.
6. Packing groceries
   o Joe will place appropriate number of items to fill bag without risk of bag breaking when carried by handles, within 3 months.

References

American Occupational Therapy Association (2011). The role of occupational therapy in end-of-life care. *American Journal of Occupational Therapy, 65*(6 Suppl.), S66-S75. doi: 10.5014/ajot.2011.65S66

American Occupational Therapy Association. (2014). Occupational therapy practice framework: Domain and process (3rd ed.). *American Journal of Occupational Therapy, 68*(1 Suppl.), S1-S48. doi: 10.5014/ajot.2014.682006

Coppard, B. M., Higgins, T., Harvey, K. D., & Padilla, R. (2012). Working with elders who have orthopedic conditions. In R. L. Padilla, S. Byers-Connon, & H. L. Lohman (Eds.), *Occupational therapy with elders: Strategies for the COTA* (3rd ed.) (pp. 299-311). Maryland Heights, MO: Elsevier Mosby.

Fike, M. L., Pendleton, K., & Hewitt, L. (2005). A telephone repairman with spinal cord injury. In K. Sladyk, & S. E. Ryan (Eds.), *Ryan's occupational therapy assistant: Principles, practice issues, and techniques* (4th ed.) (pp. 230-249). Thorofare, NJ: SLACK Incorporated.

Gateley, C. A., & Borcherding, S. (2012). *Documentation manual for occupational therapy: Writing SOAP notes* (3rd ed.). Thorofare, NJ: SLACK Incorporated.

Gillen, G. (Ed.). (2011). *Stroke rehabilitation: A function-based approach.* (3rd ed.). St. Louis, MO: Elsevier Mosby.

Gower, D., & Bowker, M. (2005). A plumber and golfer with total hip arthroplasty. In K. Sladyk, & S. E. Ryan (Eds.), *Ryan's occupational therapy assistant: Principles, practice issues, and techniques.* (4th ed.) (pp. 292-303). Thorofare, NJ: SLACK, Incorporated.

Logigian, M. (2005). A businessman with a stroke. In K. Sladyk, & S. E. Ryan (Eds.), *Ryan's occupational therapy assistant: Principles, practice issues, and techniques* (4th ed.) (pp. 318-332). Thorofare, NJ: SLACK Incorporated.

Maher, C., & Bear-Lehman, J. (2008). Orthopaedic conditions. In M. V. Radomski, & C. A. T. Latham (Eds.), *Occupational therapy for physical dysfunction* (6th ed.) (pp. 1106-1130). Baltimore, MD: Lippincott Williams & Wilkins.

Minor, M. A., & Minor, S. D. (2006). *Patient care skills* (5th ed.). Upper Saddle River, NJ: Pearson Education, Inc.

Morawski, D. L., Davis, T., & Padilla, R. (2012). Dysphagia and other eating and nutritional concerns with elders. In R. L. Padilla, S. Byers-Connon, & H. L. Lohman (Eds.), *Occupational therapy with elders: Strategies for the COTA* (3rd ed.) (pp. 251-262). Maryland Heights, MO: Elsevier Mosby.

Morawski, D. L., & Padilla, R. (2012). Working with elders who have had cerebrovascular accidents. In R. L. Padilla, S. Byers-Connon, & H. L. Lohman (Eds.), *Occupational therapy with elders: Strategies for the COTA* (3rd ed.) (pp. 263-274). Maryland Heights, MO: Elsevier Mosby.

Morreale, M. J., & Borcherding, S. (2013). *The OTA's guide to documentation: Writing SOAP notes* (3rd ed.). Thorofare, NJ: SLACK Incorporated.

Papdapoulos, E., & Deverix, B. (2013). Amputation and prosthetics. In M. B. Early (Ed.), *Physical dysfunction practice skills for the occupational therapy assistant* (3rd ed.) (pp. 654-675). St. Louis, MO: Mosby.

Peralta, A. M., Powell, S., & Plutschack, D. (2012). Working with elders who have pulmonary conditions. In R. L. Padilla, S. Byers-Connon, & H. L. Lohman (Eds.), *Occupational therapy with elders: Strategies for the COTA* (3rd ed.) (pp. 323-328). Maryland Heights, MO: Elsevier Mosby.

Spinal Cord Injury Information Pages. (2013). *Spinal cord injury functional goals.* Retrieved from www.sci-info-pages.com/function.html

Chapter 6

Developing Knowledge and Skills for Different Practice Settings

Implementing effective interventions and programs to support a client or population's occupational performance requires that OTAs in all service delivery areas demonstrate traits such as professionalism, therapeutic use of self, creative problem solving, safety awareness, and good clinical reasoning skills. Different types of settings require specialized knowledge and skills unique to those practice areas. Home care, acute care, and physical rehabilitation settings require skilled interventions that focus primarily on safety, improving specific factors/skills, and various methods to support health and engagement in areas such as ADL, IADL, and work. In the areas of mental health (behavioral health) and other activity programs (such as adult day care or assisted living), an OTA must demonstrate good behavioral observation skills, effective group leadership and mentoring skills, and the ability to select and implement appropriate activities and occupations to meet the clients' therapeutic goals. Occupational therapy in educational settings focuses on the activities and occupations that the child needs to succeed in school. Interventions may include recommendations for the classroom, such as sensory strategies, or remediation of the student's underlying weaknesses that hinder educational performance. Early intervention addresses the needs of young children with (or at risk for) developmental delay, including the contexts that hinder or support development.

The worksheets and learning activities in this chapter focus on knowledge and skills needed for various practice areas. Note that space limitations in this chapter allow for only select initial evaluation data to be presented. A "real" evaluation would include more complete information, such as the specific aspects of occupations needing assistance and the various factors, contexts, or performance skills hindering or supporting occupational performance. Answers to worksheet exercises are provided at the end of the chapter.

Contents

Morreale, M. J.
Developing Clinical Competence: A Workbook for the OTA (pp. 177-206).
© 2015 SLACK Incorporated.

Worksheet 6-1

Rehabilitation Hospital—Total Hip Replacement Goals

Mary, a 79-year-old retired secretary, had left hip replacement surgery (posterolateral approach) 5 days ago due to a hip fracture sustained in a fall. Her status for the left lower extremity is partial weight bearing. Mary's medical history includes hypertension, coronary artery disease, and hyperlipidemia. She was transferred to a rehabilitation hospital yesterday, with expected discharge to home in 10 days. Here is some additional information taken from Mary's initial evaluation report:

Living situation: Widowed and lives alone in a third floor condominium with elevator access, in an adult retirement community. There is a shower stall in one bathroom and shower/tub in a second bathroom. Client's daughter works full-time, has two children in elementary school, and lives in the next town. Her son also works full-time and lives approximately 100 miles away.

Prior level of function: Independent in all BADL and IADL. Volunteers 1 day a week at a food pantry and is active in several church groups (choir and Bible study). Client uses the town's senior citizen bus service for transportation.

Cognition: No functional deficits noted.

Upper extremity strength and range of motion: Within functional limits.

BADL: Presently unable to perform lower body dressing and bathing due to total hip precautions. Client needs moderate assistance for transfers using a rolling walker.

IADL: Dependent in household chores at this time.

Use a professional format to list four occupational therapy long-term goals for Mary.

1.

2.

3.

4.

Morreale, M. J. (2015). *Developing clinical competence: A workbook for the OTA.* Thorofare, NJ: SLACK Incorporated.

Worksheet 6-2

Home Care

1. An OTA arrives at a client's home for a scheduled occupational therapy visit. The OTA rings the doorbell several times but no one answers. The OTA should perform which primary action?

    A. Use a cell phone to call 911

    B. Use a cell phone to call the OT

    C. Use a cell phone to call the client

    D. Leave and document that no one answered the door

2. An OTA arrives at an 80-year-old female client's home for a scheduled occupational therapy visit. A person answers the door and introduces herself as the client's niece who is visiting from out of town. She tells the OTA that the client is upstairs napping. The niece asks the OTA to explain why her aunt was hospitalized recently and what her aunt needs to work on in therapy. The OTA should perform which primary action?

    A. Help the client's niece to understand the client's condition and intervention plan

    B. Wake the client up and ask for permission to talk to her niece

    C. Call the OT

    D. Call the nurse case manager

3. For clients with Medicare who require that occupational therapy services be provided at their residence, the guidelines for home care must be followed except if the client is living in which of the following settings?

    A. A relative's home

    B. An assisted living facility

    C. A skilled nursing facility

    D. A subsidized senior citizen apartment

4. An OTA is providing home care services to a client diagnosed with a shoulder fracture, hypertension, and diabetes. Today the client expresses that he is thirsty and nauseous, and the OTA observes that the client has labored breathing with a fruity breath odor. The OTA should conclude that the client is most likely at risk for which of the following?

    A. Hypoglycemia

    B. Ketoacidosis

    C. Insulin shock

    D. Orthostatic hypotension

5. A client in home care is diagnosed with chronic obstructive pulmonary disease. He exhibits deficits in endurance that limit his ability to perform IADL, such as meal preparation and laundry. The client tells the OTA he has been driving to a local restaurant for dinner most nights and to a dry cleaning establishment occasionally to get his laundry done. What is the OTA's best course of action?

    A. Work on other community mobility activities in collaboration with the OT

    B. Do not document that the client is driving because Medicare will deny home care services

    C. Document that the client no longer needs occupational therapy services

    D. Recommend outpatient occupational therapy services

Worksheet 6-2 (continued)

Home Care

6. For adult clients with Medicare or Medicaid receiving skilled home care services, which of the following outcome measures is required?

   A. OASIS

   B. DASH

   C. MDS

   D. FIM

7. According to Medicare guidelines, when a physician approves the plan of care, which of the following conditions must be met in order for an OTA to provide home care services?

   A. The OT is present during the OTA's session

   B. The physician also signs the OTA's treatment notes

   C. The OT has established the plan and provides supervision

   D. The OTA cannot provide home care for clients with Medicare

8. A client receiving home care services is recovering from bilateral lower extremity fractures. He requires assistance from his wife to use his wheelchair. When teaching wheelchair mobility in an area that lacks curb cuts, the OTA should instruct the client's wife to use which of the following methods with the wheelchair to descend a curb from the sidewalk?

   A. Approach curb with the wheelchair facing curb and tilted backward, castor wheels off the ground, and bring large wheels over the curb

   B. Approach curb with the wheelchair facing curb, lift large wheels off the ground, and bring castor wheels gently over the curb

   C. Approach curb with the wheelchair backward, ease large wheels over the curb, and tilt wheelchair backward to lift castor wheels over curb

   D. Approach curb with the wheelchair backward, tilt wheelchair forward to lift the large wheels, and ease castor wheels gently over the edge of curb

9. An OTA is working with a client in home care who has a neurological condition. As the OTA begins today's session, the client begins to exhibit a seizure. Besides obtaining medical assistance, the OTA should perform which primary action?

   A. Try to restrain the client to minimize convulsions

   B. Adjust clothing around the client's neck to loosen it

   C. Place a washcloth or wallet in client's mouth to prevent him from biting his tongue

   D. Use smelling salts and place a cool washcloth on the client's forehead

10. Which of the following statements is accurate regarding hospice services?

    A. Palliative care is provided

    B. Medicare will not reimburse for occupational and physical therapy because the client is not expected to have improved health or functional gains

    C. A physician must always certify that the client is within 1 month of death

    D. Most third-party payers will only provide reimbursement for hospice services if the diagnosis is cancer

Worksheet 6-3

Acute Care

1. A client in acute care has a Foley catheter in place. The collection bag is filled halfway with urine. When transporting the client in a wheelchair to the occupational therapy department, what should the OTA do with the catheter bag?

    A. Disconnect it

    B. Place it in the client's lap

    C. Attach it to the top of the wheelchair back support

    D. Attach it below the seat

2. An OTA client contracted a nosocomial infection. This is normally classified as which of the following?

    A. An infection that causes a coma

    B. A hospital-acquired infection

    C. An infection of the nasal cavity

    D. Nonmalignant sarcoma

3. A client recovering from congestive heart failure has an intravenous line placed in his left antecubital vein. When taking this client's vital signs, where should the OTA place the blood pressure cuff?

    A. On the client's right upper arm

    B. On the client's right forearm

    C. On the client's left upper arm

    D. On the client's left forearm

4. An OTA is working with a client who has hemiparesis and a nasogastric tube in place. Which of the following activities will most likely create the greatest risk for dislodging the tube?

    A. Active range of motion of the affected upper extremity

    B. Donning and doffing a turtleneck sweater

    C. Using a transfer belt around the client's waist

    D. Retrograde massage to the affected arm

5. When preparing to transfer a client from a hospital bed to a wheelchair using the bed rail for support, the OTA should do which of the following?

    A. Move intravenous pole in order to maintain tension at infusion site

    B. Raise the hospital bed

    C. Swing away wheelchair footrests

    D. Lower the bed rail

Worksheet 6-3 (continued)

Acute Care

6. In acute care, when does discharge planning begin for most clients?

    A. After an occupational therapy evaluation is complete

    B. Upon admission

    C. After all goals are met

    D. The day before discharge

7. During which of the following tasks is a client more likely to experience orthostatic hypotension?

    A. Elevating the foot of the bed

    B. Bilateral dowel exercises to increase shoulder range of motion

    C. Transferring sit to stand

    D. Exercising with weights

8. A client confined to bed requires maximum assistance of two people for bed mobility. Which of the following methods is likely the most useful for the OTA and nurse to use together when attempting to position the client closer to the head of the bed?

    A. Utilize a trapeze

    B. Lift the patient up by holding under his arms and legs

    C. Hold onto a sturdy cloth beneath the client

    D. Have client pull on the bed rails

9. Which of the following isolation conditions require droplet precautions?

    A. *Clostridium difficile*

    B. Tuberculosis

    C. Scabies

    D. *Streptococcus A*

10. A 50-year-old client was admitted to the intensive care unit and is unable to communicate. The client's nephew has presented documentation to the hospital staff that indicates that he is the client's health care agent. The documentation the nephew presented is most likely which of the following?

    A. Insurance card

    B. Living will

    C. Do not resuscitate form

    D. Health care proxy

Morreale, M. J. (2015). *Developing clinical competence: A workbook for the OTA.* Thorofare, NJ: SLACK Incorporated.

Worksheet 6-4

Mental Health Situations

1. A client with severe violent tendencies needs a one-on-one session to review a leisure checklist. When delegated this task, an OTA should take which of the following actions?

    A. Keep the door closed for privacy

    B. Refuse to treat the client

    C. Ask a staff member to remain in the vicinity

    D. Review the leisure checklist during an occupational therapy leisure group

2. An OTA is working with a client who is hostile and attending an anger management program. Which of the following interventions would probably be least appropriate for the OTA to implement at this time to help reduce this client's tension?

    A. Sweeping the floor

    B. Wiping tables

    C. A 15-minute walk

    D. Sanding a small wood project

3. An OTA brings a client with an eating disorder over to the craft supply closet. The OTA asks the client to choose a craft project from among the items on the shelves. The client is passive, insecure, and says repeatedly, *"I don't know what I should do"* and *"I can't decide."* What primary action should the OTA take?

    A. Use a timer to facilitate decision making

    B. Give the client a choice of two craft projects

    C. Have another client choose a project for this client

    D. Have the OTA choose a project for this client

4. An OTA in a mental health setting is leading a sensorimotor group for clients with chronic schizophrenia. Which of the following activities is most appropriate as the primary activity for this group?

    A. Writing down feelings with lively music playing in background

    B. Talking about bright colors of the rainbow

    C. Tossing and hitting a beach ball

    D. Lying on yoga mats and listening to music

5. A client in a group the OTA is leading is becoming aggressive and out of control and appears ready to hit someone. Of the following choices, the last course of action the OTA should consider taking is which of the following?

    A. Try to physically restrain the client

    B. Ask another client to go get help

    C. Talk to the client in a calm voice

    D. Remove other clients from the area

Worksheet 6-4 (continued)

Mental Health Situations

6. An OT and OTA are working on an acute psychiatric unit. They are collaborating to develop a policy and procedure manual for all the occupational therapy groups to ensure safety and meet therapeutic goals. Which of the following craft group procedures is least appropriate for the OT and OTA to include in the manual?

    A. Hand out sharps individually to clients needing them for the activity

    B. Count the number of scissors before and after the group

    C. Avoid using permanent markers and oil-based stains

    D. Give clients the autonomy to retrieve craft supplies, scissors, yarn, etc. from the occupational therapy supply closet

7. A client with schizophrenia has been attending a community mental health program but has not shown up for the past week. Today the client arrives and begins talking about how her neighbors are watching her through the TV. She also states they come in her apartment at night and move her belongings, even though her doors have a deadbolt lock. In collaboration with the OT, which of the following is most likely the best activity for the OTA to choose for this client?

    A. Writing in a journal

    B. Peeling potatoes in an IADL group

    C. Painting a picture in a crafts group

    D. Discussing feelings in an expressive group

8. During occupational therapy craft group, a client keeps picking lint off his clothing. He also keeps trying to pick lint off the other clients' clothing, despite the OTA asking him repeatedly to stop this behavior. The other clients are becoming irritated at being touched. The OTA should document the lint-picking behavior in the client's chart and describe it using which of the following terms?

    A. Obsessive behavior

    B. IADL retraining

    C. Compulsive behavior

    D. Attention to detail

9. A client attending a partial hospitalization program has a diagnosis of anxiety disorder. The client is exhibiting a panic attack, is trembling and crying, and stating she is going to die. What primary action should the OTA take?

    A. Encourage the client to take slow, deep breaths

    B. Call an ambulance

    C. Call the client's doctor

    D. Go get the OT

10. An OTA is leading a group for clients on an acute psychiatric unit who are diagnosed with depression. The group members are making items to decorate their individual hospital rooms. Of the following choices, which would likely be the most appropriate?

    A. A painted ceramic piggy bank

    B. A decorative wreath made with artificial flowers glued to a wire hanger

    C. A painted picture made with the use of stencils

    D. A colorful macramé wall hanging

Morreale, M. J. (2015). *Developing clinical competence: A workbook for the OTA.* Thorofare, NJ: SLACK Incorporated.

The Occupational Therapy Group Process

Groups in occupational therapy work toward desired outcomes, such as interaction within social norms, expression of feelings, insight into one's actions, improved coping skills and behavior, a positive self-image, and the integration of various skills needed for occupational roles. Various leaders in psychology (such as Freud, Skinner, Piaget, Erikson, etc.) and occupational therapy (such as Fidler, Mosey, Allen, etc.) have contributed important theories concerning mental functions and group process that are beyond the scope of this book. The reader is encouraged to review the primary frames of reference and models that have guided occupational therapy mental health practice. Many of these have been clearly summarized by Cole (2012), who describes the following approaches: psychodynamic, developmental, sensorimotor, cognitive-behavioral continuum, Allen's Cognitive Disabilities, and various approaches that use the Model of Human Occupation. When leading groups, the occupational therapy practitioner also needs to determine how much direction and structure the particular group requires, depending on the activity demands of the particular task, member abilities, limitations, and therapeutic goals (Cole, 2012). Anne Cronin Mosey has identified five developmental stages for group functioning, each of which addresses acquisition of particular skills: parallel groups, project groups, egocentric-cooperative groups, cooperative groups, and mature groups (Cole, 2012; Early, 2009; Tufano, 2005).

To lead occupational therapy groups effectively, an OTA, in partnership with the OT, must demonstrate the ability to design the methods and activities to meet therapeutic goals, encourage and motivate group members, set limits, recognize defense mechanisms, handle problem behaviors, use therapeutic qualities and communication skills (i.e., sensitivity, genuineness, attending, empathy, limited self-disclosure, modeling of appropriate behavior, etc.), understand individual and group member roles, and determine capacities and limitations of members (Cole, 2012; Early, 2009; Tufano, 1997, 2003, 2005). Cole (2012) describes, at length, seven steps for effective group leadership in occupational therapy, which she adapted from Pfeiffer and Jones' *Reference Guide to Handbooks and Annuals* (1977). Cole's Seven-Step Format for Group Leadership, briefly summarized in the following text, is very useful for highest level groups and can also be modified to meet other groups' needs (Cole, 2012).

Cole's Seven-Step Groups (2012)

1. Introduction—The start of a group should include an introduction of the occupational therapy practitioner and participants, along with a warm-up to set the mood and encourage attention. The leader explains the group's purpose, outlines the session, and delineates the time frame and expectations.

2. Activity—The leader chooses an activity designed to meet therapeutic goals. The activity is based on multiple factors, such as time constraints, the members' mental and physical abilities, and the leader's skill/knowledge. Other considerations for the activity include adaptations needed; amount of intended structure, creativity, or social interaction; and the specific method of instruction to implement the task.

3. Sharing—Group members show their work or explain their feelings. The group leader encourages participation and acknowledges each person verbally or nonverbally.

4. Processing—Group members express their feelings about the group experience and interactions with peers and leader. The underlying group dynamics may be explored.

5. Generalizing—The leader summarizes the learning aspects and general cognitive principles ascertained through the group process.

6. Application—The identified principles are applied to life situations. Practical methods are discussed and the leader may provide limited self-disclosure to model solutions.

7. Summary—Important aspects of the group are emphasized briefly, such as goals and knowledge achieved. The leader notes changes of behavior, acknowledges and thanks members for their participation.

Learning Activity 6-1: Eating Disorders

The facility you are working at is starting a new program for young adults with eating disorders. You are collaborating with the OT to develop an ADL group that will be implemented in this program. Consider occupational therapy discussion topics or activities relating to areas such as dressing, eating, shopping for food or clothing, health maintenance, etc. Choose a particular BADL or IADL and use Cole's Seven-Step Format for Group Leadership (2012) to help plan an entire group session for 6 clients. Determine how much time you will allocate for each stage of this group. Realize that actual activities used in a treatment program will depend upon the specific approach or frame of reference that the OT (and team) determines is appropriate for that setting and particular group of clients.

Frame of reference for activity: _____

Occupation to be addressed: _____

Activity: _____

Length of group:_____

1. Introduction: Time allocated: _____minutes
    - What specific words or actions will you use to greet the members and warm-up the group? How will you outline the group's purpose and expectations?

2. Activity: Time allocated: _____minutes
    - What specific activity will the group do? How and where will you set up the activity and position the clients? List the activity demands, such as equipment or supplies needed, specific content of any worksheets/ written materials used, method of instruction, sequence of steps, etc.

3. Sharing: Time allocated: _____minutes
    - What would you like the members to share? What will you ask and do to encourage member participation?

4. Processing: Time allocated: _____minutes
    - What will you ask or say to encourage member participation? What aspects of the group process will you focus on?

5. Generalizing: Time allocated: _____minutes
    - What concepts do you want the clients to learn?

6. Application: Time allocated: _____minutes
    - How can this experience be applied to other life situations? What limited self-disclosure might you offer?

7. Summary: Time allocated: _____minutes
    - What will you say to summarize and provide a closing for the group?

Adapted from Cole, M.B. (2012). *Group dynamics in occupational therapy: The theoretical basis and practice application of group intervention* (4th ed). Thorofare, NJ: SLACK Incorporated.

Worksheet 6-5

Social Skills Group—Picnic

Imagine you are leading an occupational therapy social skills group for clients with high cognitive abilities who have been allowed to go on a supervised community outing. The varied diagnoses of the group members include anxiety disorder, mood disorder, obsessive-compulsive disorder, and borderline personality disorder. After collaboration with the OT, you have determined that the group should plan and prepare a picnic lunch over the course of several sessions. Food items may be obtained from the facility's food service department (with 24 hours notice), and the facility has a transportation service. Consider some ways in which you can facilitate interaction among the group members for this occupation. For each conversation starter idea you list for this egocentric-cooperative group, indicate a practical method (an activity) for implementing that discussion. Here is an example:

1. Topic:

   Encourage group members to determine a common menu, taking into account likes, dislikes, food allergies, dietary restrictions, and availability of items.

   Possible activity/method:

   Group leader provides each client with a worksheet listing 10 food choices. Clients number them in order of priority from 1 to 10.

   or

   Each client is provided with a list of all available food items to check off or circle one desired item in each category (i.e., beverage, dessert).

   Worksheet answers can be listed on a white board or flip chart. Group members discuss answers and decide on menu. Consider factors such as decision making, cooperation, and compromise.

2. Topic:

   Activity/method:

3. Topic:

   Activity/method:

4. Topic:

   Activity/method:

Morreale, M. J. (2015). *Developing clinical competence: A workbook for the OTA*. Thorofare, NJ: SLACK Incorporated.

Worksheet 6-5 (continued)
Social Skills Group—Picnic

5. Topic:

    Activity/method:

6. Topic:

    Activity/method:

7. Topic:

    Activity/method:

8. Topic:

    Activity/method:

9. Topic:

    Activity/method:

10. Topic:

    Activity/method:

Learning Activity 6-2: Four Current Events Groups

Imagine you are leading four separate occupational therapy current events groups (and collaborating with an OT when required by law for that setting). For each of the groups, choose a recent, interesting article from a newspaper to discuss with the group members. Pick a different article for each group, considering the therapeutic needs of the particular group. For each article, develop eight open-ended questions you might use as conversation starters to facilitate interaction among the group members. Determine the therapeutic purpose for each of the groups and incorporate occupational therapy group process skills. Indicate the lessons that members can learn from discussing the article and application to life situations.

For example, you might ask the group questions such as:

- What is your opinion about that?
- What do you think will happen next?
- Why do you agree or disagree with that proposed law?
- Why is that important?
- What are the pros and cons of that?
- Can you describe a similar experience you had?
- What would you have done in the same situation?
- Why do you think he committed that crime?
- Do you think the punishment fits the crime? Why or why not?

1. **Inpatient Behavioral Health Unit: Chemical Dependency/Alcohol Abuse**
    You are an OTA working on an acute inpatient behavioral health unit. The group participants have high cognitive abilities and are diagnosed with chemical dependency or alcohol abuse.

    Topic of article:_____

    Purpose of group:_____

    General principles to be discussed/applied:_____

    _____

    _____

    Conversation starter questions:

    A.

    B.

    C.

    D.

    E.

    F.

    G.

    H.

2. Senior Citizen Program

You are an activity leader for a local senior citizen day program.

Topic of article:_____

Purpose of group:_____

General principles to be discussed/applied:_____

_____

_____

Conversation starter questions:

A.

B.

C.

D.

E.

F.

G.

H.

3. Social Day Program: Developmental Disability

You are an activity leader working in a social day program for young adults who live with their families. Each participant has a developmental disability with mild to moderate intellectual impairment. However, each participant has functional verbal skills.

Topic of article:_____

Purpose of group:_____

General principles to be discussed/applied:_____

_____

_____

Conversation starter questions:

A.

B.

C.

D.

E.

F.

G.

H.

4. **School Program: Bullying**

You are an OTA working in a school program designed to prevent bullying and are leading a small group of middle-school students.

Topic of article:_____

Purpose of group:_____

General principles to be discussed/applied:_____

_____

_____

Conversation starter questions:

A.

B.

C.

D.

E.

F.

G.

H.

Worksheet 6-6

Social Skills Group—Collage Craft

Pretend you are leading an occupational therapy social skills group for clients who have high cognitive abilities and various mental health conditions, such as mood disorders, anxiety, and substance abuse. After collaboration with the OT, you have determined that the group members should work together to make one big collage. List 10 possible ways to facilitate interaction among group members as they are making the collage.

Here is an example:

1. *Group participants must decide on a common theme such as "Happiness" or "Family."*

2.

3.

4.

5.

6.

7.

8.

9.

10.

11.

Learning Activity 6-3: Interventions in Mental Health— Frames of Reference

For each of the following occupational therapy groups, list the frame of reference you will utilize and three activities appropriate for **adult clients with depression**. For these exercises, assume that you have collaborated with the OT.

Activity Group

Frame of reference:_____

List three craft projects that the client can choose from and explain why you chose each craft. For example, is the craft a quick-success project, or does it allow the client to express emotions? You will also need to decide if tasks will be performed individually or as a collaborative effort.

1. _____

2. _____

3. _____

According to the frame of reference, this particular activity was chosen because_____

_____

_____

Expressive Group

Frame of reference:_____

List three discussion topics or activities for this group and explain why you chose each one. For example, does the activity facilitate interpersonal skills or exploration of feelings?

1. _____

2. _____

3. _____

According to the frame of reference, this particular activity was chosen because_____

_____

_____

IADL Group

Frame of reference:_____

List three possible IADL activities for this group and explain why you chose each one. For example, does the activity facilitate role performance or promote healthy habits?

1. _____

2. _____

3. _____

According to the frame of reference, this particular activity was chosen because_____

_____

_____

Learning Activity 6-4: More Interventions in Mental Health

For each of the following occupational therapy groups, list three activities appropriate for **young adults diagnosed with substance abuse**. You will also need to decide if tasks will be performed individually or as a collaborative effort. For this exercise, assume that you have collaborated with the OT.

Activity Group

Frame of reference:_____

List three craft projects that the client can choose from and explain why you chose each craft. For example, is the craft a quick-success project, or does it allow the client to express emotions?

    1. _____

    2. _____

    3. _____

According to the frame of reference, this particular activity was chosen because_____

_____

_____

Expressive Group

Frame of reference:_____

List three discussion topics or activities for this group and explain why you chose each one. For example, does the activity encourage client to express emotions or teach coping strategies?

    1. _____

    2. _____

    3. _____

According to the frame of reference, this particular activity was chosen because_____

_____

_____

Leisure Group

Frame of reference:_____

List three possible activities for this group and explain why you chose each one. For example, does the activity develop leisure skills or help alleviate stress?

    1. _____

    2. _____

    3. _____

According to the frame of reference, this particular activity was chosen because_____

_____

_____

Five-Stage Group Format Designed by Ross

Ross (1997) designed a Five-Stage Group format based on neurophysiological principles for clients who have low cognitive or social abilities, developmental disability, nonverbal/limited communication, or behavioral problems (i.e., hostility, acting out). Ross advocates a structured progression of sensory stimulation as a means to motivate the group, improve behavior and social skills, and help members process and organize information. Desired responses are elicited through sensory activities (i.e., vestibular, tactile, proprioceptive, visual, etc.) and the activities' effect on the central nervous system (Ross, 1997). Ross's Five-Stage Group format is briefly summarized below (Ross, 1997):

- Stage 1: Orientation—Introductions and a simple 1-minute activity (i.e., handle simple instruments, pass around items, use scents, noisemakers, etc.) to increase alertness, facilitate calmness and relaxation, and provide sensory stimulation.
- Stage 2: Movement—This stage consists of motor activities, such as reaching, walking, hopping, dance, or activities using props such as a parachute, ball, ribbon wand, scarves, hoops, etc.
- Stage 3: Visual-motor perceptual activities—Consists of more challenging tasks, such as puzzles, activities addressing body parts (i.e., Simon Says), and eye-hand coordination (i.e., golf putting, plastic bowling).
- Stage 4: Cognitive stimulation and function—Activities such as stories, short poems, discussions, memory and guessing games, etc. are used to increase communication and help organize thoughts and behavior.
- Stage 5: Closing the session—A brief, familiar routine is used to signal the end of the session and provide positivity (i.e., a song, snack, hold hands, etc.).

Learning Activity 6-5: Assisted Living Facility

Imagine you are an activity leader for the Alzheimer's unit in an assisted living facility. You would like to provide the residents with meaningful opportunities to reminisce, handle objects, engage in familiar activities, and socialize. Use Ross's Five-Stage Group format (1997) to design a group session. Create an activity box relating to a familiar occupation and plan the group around this theme. Keep in mind any safety concerns or dietary restrictions. An example of an activity box and relevant group activities for a session are provided.

Occupation	IADL: Baking	
Activity box contents	Egg beater, wooden spoon, spatula, small muffin tin, sifter, plastic measuring cups, measuring spoons, small rolling pin, cookie cutters	
Stage 1	Greeting and introduction Smell spices used in baking (i.e., vanilla, cinnamon, ginger)	
Stage 2	Roll out prepared sugar cookie dough with a rolling pin	
Stage 3	Cut out cookies with a cookie cutter and place on a cookie sheet	
Stage 4	Each group member selects a kitchen item to handle and name Reminisce about baking, favorite desserts	
Stage 5	Closing remarks, provide a snack that clients are allowed to eat (i.e., cookies)	

Morreale, M. J. (2015). *Developing clinical competence: A workbook for the OTA.* Thorofare, NJ: SLACK Incorporated.

Worksheet 6-7

Skilled Nursing Facility

1. Which of the following ADL impairments is typically one of the earliest symptoms an individual may exhibit as an early sign of Alzheimer's disease?

   A. Incontinence

   B. Forgetting how to shave or brush teeth

   C. Forgetting how to operate a car

   D. Difficulty with remembering names or appointments

2. An OTA is working with a client, Stella, diagnosed with Alzheimer's disease and functioning at Allen Cognitive Level 3. The client is recovering from a thoracic compression fracture and appears to have back pain. Stella requires assistance for all ADL and often asks when her mother, who is deceased, will be coming to visit. When assisting the client with upper and lower body dressing, which of the following methods is probably the least useful for this client?

   A. Teaching use of a sock assist to don socks

   B. Using validation technique

   C. Using chaining technique to don a shirt

   D. Using task breakdown

3. Mary, a client with dementia, cannot remember to ask staff for assistance when she wants to get out of her wheelchair. She is at risk for falls due to poor balance and inability to remember to use her walker. Mary also has poor fine-motor skills. Which primary intervention should an OTA suggest as an alternative to a restraint while Mary sits in her wheelchair?

   A. Seat belt with buckle

   B. Vest restraint

   C. Seat alarm

   D. Lap board

4. An OTA in a skilled nursing facility is working with a client who exhibits left neglect. Which of the following activities is least appropriate for the OTA to do?

   A. Implement a symmetrical bilateral activity

   B. Implement an asymmetrical bilateral activity

   C. Apply lotion to the client's left arm

   D. When leaving, the OTA should state that the call bell is on the client's left side

5. An OTA is working with a client with dementia functioning at Allen Cognitive Level 2. The client is exhibiting agitation and keeps asking when her husband will arrive. The OTA knows that the client's spouse has been deceased for 10 years. Which of the following methods would probably be the least effective for an OTA to use with this client?

   A. Reality orientation

   B. Therapeutic fib

   C. Redirect attention

   D. Validation

Morreale, M. J. (2015). *Developing clinical competence: A workbook for the OTA.* Thorofare, NJ: SLACK Incorporated.

Worksheet 6-8

Pediatrics—Early Intervention

1. Which of the following choices is correct regarding the developmental sequence of prehension from earlier to later?

   A. Raking grasp, radial digital grasp, inferior pincer grasp

   B. Raking grasp, palmar grasp, developmental scissors grasp

   C. Radial digital grasp, radial palmar grasp, three-jaw chuck

   D. Inferior pincer grasp, developmental scissors grasp, radial digital grasp

2. Under the Individuals With Disabilities Education Act (IDEA), the term *least restrictive environment* refers to which of the following conditions?

   A. Minimizing clutter in the home to allow for motor development

   B. Avoiding the use of restraints for positioning

   C. A therapy room that has adequate space for required therapy tasks, such as sensory integration equipment

   D. Placing atypical children in settings with typical children

3. To best facilitate bilateral integration for a 7-month-old infant who is able to sit unsupported but does not demonstrate spontaneous use of the left upper extremity, an OTA should place the child in which position?

   A. Standing to push a toy shopping cart

   B. Supine to reach for a mobile

   C. Right side-lying to hold a stuffed animal

   D. Ring sitting to pick up 1-inch blocks

4. Which of the following clients would not currently be eligible for early intervention services under Part C of IDEA?

   A. A 3-month-old infant born with low birth weight to a mother who abuses alcohol

   B. A 6-year-old child diagnosed with Duchenne muscular dystrophy

   C. A 1.5-year-old child diagnosed with failure to thrive

   D. A 30-month-old child diagnosed with lead poisoning

5. An OTA at a preschool is working with child diagnosed with a developmental delay. The OTA asks the child to identify alphabet letters written on a blackboard and painted on blocks. The OTA also has the child pick out magnetic letters to spell the child's name. The underlying prewriting skill that is not being specifically addressed with these tasks is which of the following?

   A. Visual closure

   B. Form constancy

   C. Visual memory

   D. Visual discrimination

Morreale, M. J. (2015). *Developing clinical competence: A workbook for the OTA*. Thorofare, NJ: SLACK Incorporated.

Worksheet 6-9

Pediatrics—School Setting

1. An OTA was delegated the task of observing a first-grade student, Olivia, to ascertain the prehension pattern that Olivia uses for writing. The OTA observes that, as Olivia is completing a homework assignment, she is holding the pencil in her right hand and using a static quadrupod grasp. The OTA should inform the OT that Olivia is using what kind of grasp?

   A. Primitive

   B. Transitional

   C. Reflexive

   D. Mature

2. Steven is a second-grade student who has decreased pinch strength in his dominant right hand. As a result, he exhibits difficulty with handwriting and reports his hand gets tired. Steven's Individualized Education Program (IEP) delineates that an occupational therapy consultative model will be used to address these deficits. In order to implement the IEP, which of the following actions should the OTA take?

   A. Work with Steven directly in the occupational therapy room to address fine-motor skills using media such as therapy putty and clothespins

   B. Work with Steven directly in the classroom to address fine-motor skills using media such as clay and a pegboard

   C. Suggest to the teacher that Steven use clay at play time and 1-inch pom-poms to erase a whiteboard

   D. Co-treat with the PT to improve Steven's fine-motor skills more quickly

3. In a school setting, which of the following would not likely be a goal established in an IEP for a 14-year-old female student diagnosed with autism and dyspraxia?

   A. Ability to get from one class to another on time

   B. Ability to apply make-up independently

   C. Ability to manage feminine hygiene independently

   D. Ability to select and insert proper denomination of coins to use a cafeteria vending machine

4. An OTA is working in a school setting with Evan, a second-grade student who exhibits poor attention and fidgets frequently while seated at his desk. Which of the following is least appropriate for the OTA to recommend to Evan's teacher?

   A. Have Evan sit directly under the bright overhead lighting to allow him to see better and improve concentration

   B. Have Evan use headphones to reduce ambient noise during independent tasks

   C. Have Evan help move a stack of books or classroom furniture

   D. Allow Evan to use a "fidget," such as a small squeeze ball, when seated at his desk

5. An OTA is working in a school setting with a 12-year-old student named Daisy who is diagnosed with a developmental disability. During today's occupational therapy session, Daisy begins to sob and states that her classmates are saying mean things about her on the Internet. Besides informing the OT, what primary action should the OTA should take?

   A. Tell Daisy she is overreacting and should ignore the other student's comments

   B. Call the other children's parents

   C. Notify the police

   D. Ask Daisy for specific examples

Answers to Worksheets

Worksheet 6-1: Rehabilitation Hospital—Total Hip Replacement Goals

Resources for goal writing: Gateley & Borcherding, 2012; Morreale & Borcherding, 2013

Goals need to specify a time frame, measurable criteria, and delineate a desired client behavior relating to function. Goals should reflect what the client needs to achieve, not what the occupational therapy practitioner will do as interventions. Here are some suggested goals for this client. Realize that different settings or practice areas may use slightly different formats or terminology, as shown in the various examples that follow. Of course, the actual goals and time frames may be different for a real client.

1. Client will complete lower body dressing with modified independence and adhere to all total hip precautions by expected discharge in 10 days.

    or

    By expected discharge in 10 days, client will don lower body garments independently using adaptive equipment and adhere to hip precautions.

2. Client will perform lower body bathing with modified independence and adhere to all total hip precautions by expected discharge in 10 days.

    or

    While seated on a tub bench and adhering to hip precautions, client will bathe lower body independently by expected discharge in 10 days.

3. Client will demonstrate ability to heat items in microwave independently while using wheeled walker in kitchen, and adhere to all total hip precautions by expected discharge in 10 days.

4. In order to manage grooming tasks independently, client will demonstrate 8 minutes standing tolerance at sink using rolling walker within 10 days.

5. Client will complete toilet transfers with modified independence (using wheeled walker, elevated seat, and grab bar) and adhere to all total hip precautions by expected discharge in 10 days.

6. In order to manage IADL more independently, client will increase bilateral upper extremity strength by ½ muscle grade by expected discharge in 10 days.

7. Client will demonstrate ability to prepare a simple stove-top meal (i.e., eggs, soup) while standing with walker with contact guard assistance within 1 week.

Worksheet 6-2: Home Care

1. C. The client may be in the bathroom or might not have heard the doorbell, so the primary course of action would be to try and reach him by phone. If there is still no answer, the OTA should follow agency policy, such as contacting the OT and nurse case manager and document the situation.

2. B. An OTA must always adhere to the Health Insurance Portability and Accountability Act (HIPAA) guidelines. As the OTA must wake up the client for therapy, the OTA should ask the client for permission to discuss the client's medical information with her niece. The client may or may not want it disclosed.

3. C. According to Centers for Medicare & Medicaid Services ([CMS] 2003b) guidelines, A, B, and D may be considered as the client's residence. If a client is in a skilled nursing facility, regulations for that setting would apply instead.

4. B. These may be symptoms of hyperglycemia, which can cause ketoacidosis (diabetic coma), and is a very serious condition (George, 2013; Oakes, 2010).

5. D. If the client is able to drive around the community independently, he may no longer ethically meet the Medicare criteria for being homebound and this should be discussed with the health team (CMS, 2003a). The client may still benefit from therapy to address his ADL deficits and can be referred to an outpatient clinic.

6. A. The Outcome Assessment Information Set (OASIS) is required (CMS, 2012), although the health practitioner may choose to utilize any additional assessments such as the Disability of Arm, Shoulder, and Hand (DASH) and Functional Independence Measure (FIM). The Minimum Data Set (MDS) is used in skilled nursing facilities.

7. C. Medicare guidelines for occupational therapy (CMS, 2011) require that an OT perform the assessment and establish, manage, and supervise the plan of care. The OT must also perform client reassessments at specified intervals. An OT does not have to be physically present when an OTA implements a delegated treatment session in between those intervals. While the physician must certify changes in the plan of care, there is no requirement that the physician sign treatment notes.

8. C. Fairchild, 2013.

9. B. During a seizure, do not restrain the client or place objects in the client's mouth. Adjust clothing around the neck to help keep the client from having a restricted airway and call for medical help (George, 2013; Oakes, 2010).

10. A. Typically, a client must be terminally ill with a prognosis of 6 months or less to receive hospice care, which a physician must certify. In addition to cancer diagnoses, benefits are provided for other terminal conditions, such as congestive heart failure, non-Alzheimer's dementia, failure to thrive, chronic kidney disease, etc. (CMS, 2013).

Worksheet 6-3: Acute Care

1. D. The urine collection bag should be below the bladder level to avoid backflow (Fairchild, 2013; George, 2013).

2. B. A nosocomial infection is a generic term for a hospital-acquired infection, which can include hepatitis B, *Clostridium difficile*, and other conditions. The more recent term, *health care-associated infections*, is now being utilized to reflect all areas of health practice (Siegel, Rhinehart, Jackson, Chiarello, & the Healthcare Infection Control Practices Advisory Committee, 2007).

3. A. Avoid placing the cuff above the intravenous insertion site (Fairchild, 2013).

4. B. The tube is inserted through the nose. Care must be taken so that donning and doffing an overhead sweater does not tug or pull at the tube.

5. C. The intravenous line should not be taut. The bed should be lowered so that the client's feet can reach the floor when seated on the edge of the bed for safety. Wheelchair footrests should be in the swing away position or removed. If a client is using bed rails to aid in transfers, the rails should be locked in the up position.

6. B. Lengths of stay in acute care are often very short. As soon as the client is admitted, the team members consider if the client will be returning home, will need continued rehabilitation at another facility (e.g., skilled nursing facility, rehabilitation hospital), or will transfer to a different setting (e.g., relative's home). This will help give the discharge planner time to coordinate the transfer or any discharge recommendations. In acute care, not all clients will need or receive occupational therapy.

7. C. For some clients, sudden postural changes may cause the client's blood pressure to drop significantly and may cause lightheadedness or fainting.

8. C. A draw sheet under the client makes it easier for staff to move and position a client in bed who requires much assistance. Lifting a client up by the arms and legs poses greater risk for injury to both the client and health workers. While the client can attempt to assist by pulling up using a trapeze or bed rails, they are not the best option in this situation.

9. D. In terms of isolation procedures, *Streptococcus* A requires droplet precautions, tuberculosis requires airborne precautions, and scabies and *Clostridium difficile* require contact precautions (Siegel et al., 2007).

10. D. A health care proxy designates an individual who can make health care decisions on one's behalf in case of incapacitation.

Worksheet 6-4: Mental Health Situations

1. C. For safety reasons, the OTA should keep the door open and ensure that a staff member is in the vicinity in case the client becomes aggressive.

2. A. A client can use a mop or broom as a weapon (Early, 2009).

3. B. While a timer could possibly work, it is not the best option as it could create more stress for the client and lessen feelings of self-control. A full closet of craft options may be too overwhelming for this client, so minimizing the choices to two options would be appropriate to facilitate decision making. Having others choose the project would not allow for the client to experience any self-control or decision making.

4. C. The only choice consisting of a gross-motor activity is the beach ball activity.

5. A. If a client is becoming out of control, it is best for the OTA to call for help, talk in a calm voice, and remove other clients from the area. Physically restraining a client should be avoided and used only as a last resort (Early, 2009).

6. D. To help ensure safety, an occupational therapy practitioner must carefully keep track of sharps and other hazardous objects, such as string and yarn. Items with fumes (e.g., stains, dyes) can also be dangerous (Early, 2009).

7. B. A client experiencing hallucinations would benefit from activities that are structured (i.e., familiar tasks to help the client to maintain appropriate focus [Early, 2009]).

8. C. The client is acting on his obsessive thoughts and demonstrating compulsive behavior.

9. A. An OTA should always use clinical judgment to distinguish between a true medical emergency versus the client's pattern of panic attacks, and take action accordingly. For a panic attack, generally the first course of action is to encourage the client to take slow, deep breaths to help the anxiety to pass.

10. C. A wire hanger, glass, and cords can be used by a client to harm self or others (Early, 2009).

Worksheet 6-5: Social Skills Group—Picnic

In general, the OTA should facilitate positive interaction among group members; provide necessary feedback regarding appropriate and inappropriate language and behavior exhibited; and provide opportunities for socialization, leisure, and learning, such as application of the group experience to life and strategies (Cole, 2012). Here are some practical suggestions to facilitate interaction among group members for this picnic task. Realize these are only suggestions and may not be appropriate for each group of clients. Actual implementation and choice of a particular method or activity will depend upon the specific approach or frame of reference that the OT (and team) determines is appropriate for a particular group of clients.

1. Topic: Encourage group members to determine a common menu, taking into account likes, dislikes, food allergies, dietary restrictions, and availability of items.

    Possible activity/method:

    ‣ Group leader provides each client with a worksheet listing 10 food choices. Clients number them in order of priority from 1 to 10.

        or

    ‣ Each client is provided with a list of all available food items to check off or circle one desired item in each category (i.e., beverage, dessert).

    Worksheet answers can be listed on a white board or flip chart. Group members discuss answers and decide on menu. Consider factors such as decision making, cooperation, and compromise.

2. Topic: Group members can discuss feeling/attitudes toward picnics or going outdoors, considering past experiences and anticipation of task.

    Possible activity/method:

    ‣ Have client anonymously write a word or phrase on an index card describing his or her feelings toward the upcoming picnic activity, such as *fun, anxious, relaxing, boring*, etc., and place it in a basket for discussion.

        or

    ‣ Worksheet: Each client circles or checks off from a list describing how the client is feeling regarding the upcoming picnic, then discusses.

3. Topic: Once menu has been decided, group members must come up with a list of all items needed for the picnic.

    Possible activity/method:

    ‣ Group leader (or member) writes down member suggestions on a large flip chart or white board. Can list by categories (specific food items/condiments, eating and serving equipment, recreational items, etc.).

4. Topic: Group members must determine time frames for preparatory tasks (i.e., order food 2 days prior, bake cupcakes 1 day prior, make sandwiches morning of the picnic).

    Possible activity/method:

    ‣ Group leader (or member) writes down list of steps and member suggestions on a large flip chart or white board. Discuss factors such as organization and time management.

5. Topic: Group members must decide on a picnic location within a certain radius.

    Possible activity/method:

    ▸ Group leader provides each client with a worksheet listing five choices of locations. Clients are asked to number them in order of priority from 1 to 5 and then discuss and decide on location. The pros and cons can be written on a flip chart or white board.

6. Topic: Group members should discuss alternatives if it rains.

    Possible activity/method:

    ▸ Worksheet: Clients write down two alternative solutions or choose from a list of possible alternatives. Member suggestions can be written on a flip chart or white board for discussion.

7. Topic: Group members can plan for other recreational activities at picnic site, such as sedentary or active leisure tasks.

    Possible method/activity:

    ▸ Each member fills out leisure inventory/checklist. Clients choose two items to suggest to the rest of group or write them on index cards and place in a basket for discussion. Consider factors of cooperation and compromise.

8. Topic: Group members must plan how food items will be prepared (i.e., Will the dietary department provide premade sandwiches? Will each person prepare his or her own sandwich? Will each member prepare a component of the meal for everyone? Will the group bake a batch of cookies together? etc.).

    Possible method/activity:

    ▸ List options on flip chart or white board, discuss, and decide. Consider factors such as food safety, decision making, cooperation.

9. Topic: Cooperation/compromise.

    Possible method/activity:

    ▸ Perform a meal preparation task, such as baking cookies or preparing a salad, for which group members must work cooperatively and actually have to share kitchen tools, spices, plastic wrap, etc.

10. Topic: Favorite recipes (their own or someone else's).

    Possible method/activity:

    ▸ Members can look up recipes for various picnic foods or bring a familiar recipe to share with the group. Group members can discuss or teach their own method/recipe for the meal components, such as a favorite recipe for cookies or potato salad.

        or

    ▸ Members can use a worksheet to list one or more favorite homemade foods and answer questions, such as if this food is healthy/unhealthy, a special treat, a childhood favorite, holiday related, how often it was available, etc.

11. Topic: Group members must decide how food will be packed (i.e., individual boxed lunches or shared platters of food).

    Possible method/activity:

    ▸ List options on flip chart or white board and discuss. Consider factors such as food safety, decision making, cooperation.

12. Topic: Group members can discuss/critique the prepared food, picnic outing experience, and interaction with peers.

    Possible method/activity:

    ▸ Have each client anonymously write a word or phrase on an index card describing his or her feelings/attitude toward the picnic activity, such as *fun, anxious, relaxing, stupid*, etc., and place in a basket for discussion.

        or

    ▸ Worksheet: Each client circles or checks off from a list describing how the client felt regarding the picnic and then discusses his or her choices.

or

- ▸ Worksheet: Rate each category (i.e., food, location, overall experience, etc.) on a scale from 0 to 10, then discuss.

13. Topic: Group members can discuss feeling/attitudes toward food (i.e., emotional eating, comfort foods, healthy/unhealthy foods).

Possible activity/method:

- ▸ Worksheet: Have client write down specific foods that he or she usually eats in various designated situations, such as when feeling stressed, watching TV, needing energy, as a reward/treat, etc.

Worksheet 6-6: Social Skills Group—Collage Craft

The OTA should encourage positive interaction among group members and provide feedback regarding appropriate and inappropriate language and behavior exhibited. Here are some suggestions to facilitate interaction among group members as they are making the collage.

1. Group participants must decide on a common theme such as "Happiness" or "Family." They may be provided with a list to choose from if more structure is needed.
2. Ask a group member who has made a collage before to teach others how to do the craft.
3. Limit materials so that clients will have to share (e.g., only one bottle of glue).
4. Ask group members to divide up the activity demands and decide who will do what aspects of the project (i.e., one person has to find magazines on the unit, another person has to clear and set up the work surface with newspapers).
5. Ask group members to explain why they chose the pictures they did.
6. Ask group members to comment on others' pictures.
7. Group members can be asked to collaboratively decide on picture placement.
8. Ask group members to decide on other possible art materials to decorate the collage (e.g., glitter, foam letters).
9. Ask group members to discuss or critique the finished product.
10. Create some situations to address frustration tolerance or facilitate problem-solving or decision-making skills, such as creating time constraints, running out of some materials, and establishing additional criteria (i.e., cannot use a picture of a person or all words must have red letters).
11. Ask group members to discuss their feelings regarding participation in this activity.
12. Ask group members to decide where to place the finished collage.

Worksheet 6-7: Skilled Nursing Facility

1. D. Memory difficulty is an early sign for people with Alzheimer's. While an individual in the early stages may still be able to operate a car, a big concern is that *the person may not be able to do this safely*. The person may have problems with following the rules of the road, spatial orientation, reaction time, or may easily get lost and create significant safety concerns. Family education and other measures (i.e., take away keys, disable car) should be put in place to help keep an unsafe person from operating a motor vehicle (Alzheimer's Association, 2009).

2. A. A client functioning at Allen Cognitive Level 3 has poor problem-solving skills and diminished capacity for new learning, particularly when a device is unfamiliar, such as a sock assist. For this client, the OTA's time would probably be better spent working on other aspects of dressing in which the client can better participate.

3. C. A seat alarm would not restrain Mary, but would alert staff if she begins to stand. As Mary has poor fine-motor skills, a seat belt with buckle and a lap board are considered restraints if the client is unable to open or remove them.

4. D. For clients with unilateral neglect, it is useful for an OTA to incorporate activities that involve having the client use both upper extremities, such as using a rolling pin (symmetrical task) or holding toothpaste in one hand and applying it to a toothbrush held in the other hand (asymmetrical task). Applying lotion to the neglected side can help bring attention to it. *The call bell should always be placed where the client can attend to it if needed.* In this situation, it should be placed to Mary's right side, not the left.

5.   A. A client functioning at Allen Cognitive Level 2 has severe cognitive impairment. Reality orientation would not be effective. Answers B, C, and D are techniques that can be utilized with a caring approach to minimize the client's apparent emotional discomfort (Hellen & Padilla, 2012).

Worksheet 6-8: Pediatrics—Early Intervention

1.   A. Edwards, Buckland, & McCoy-Powlen, 2002.

2.   D. Part C provides services to eligible children under the age of 3 (Küpper, 2012; U.S. Department of Education, n.d.).

3.   C. To best facilitate use of both hands, placing the child lying on the right side would limit motion of the uninvolved arm and encourage the child to use the affected left arm together to hold the stuffed toy. Reaching for a mobile and picking up blocks does not involve simultaneous use of both hands, although they could be used to encourage use of the involved arm. At 7 months, the child would not yet have the ability to walk.

4.   B. Under Part C of IDEA, early intervention services are provided from birth up to age 3 for children with, or at risk for, a disability and their families. However, under IDEA Part B, related services and special education can be extended to age 21 (Küpper, 2012; U.S. Department of Education, n.d.).

5.   A. Visual closure involves the identification of a letter or figure when it is incomplete. This is a skill needed to form letters when writing, but in this situation the letters are already complete (Pendzick & Rockwell, 2009).

Worksheet 6-9: Pediatrics—School Setting

1.   B. Edwards et al., 2002.

2.   C. Occupational therapy practitioners using a consultative model provide direct recommendations to the teacher and other education staff to implement with a particular student, such as strategies or activities the student would benefit from in the classroom. A direct service model provides designated therapy services to the child individually or in a group, such as exercises for postural control, gross and fine-motor tasks, sensory integration activities, etc. The two models are not always mutually exclusive (Steva, 2010).

3.   B. Goals in an IEP must relate to the skills a student needs to function within the school environment. Toileting skills, feminine hygiene, ability to get to class, and cafeteria functions, such as carrying a tray, purchasing lunch/snacks (i.e., using a school vending machine), are all related to the educational setting. While the student may desire to be able to apply make-up independently, it is not an educationally related task.

4.   A. A child with poor attention would benefit more from calming strategies, such as dim lighting and answers B, C, and D (Gallagher, 2005).

5.   D. Harassment, intimidation, and bullying (HIB) is a serious matter that should not be taken lightly. An OTA working in a school setting has a duty to report such behavior to help ensure the child's safety and emotional well-being. The OTA should ask the child about the general nature of the comments (i.e., teasing versus direct threat of bodily harm) and follow the protocol that the school district has in place for handling these situations.

References

Alzheimer's Association. (2009). *10 early signs and symptoms of Alzheimer's*. Retrieved from www.alz.org/alzheimers_disease_10_signs_of_alzheimers.asp

Centers for Medicare & Medicaid Services. (2003a). *Medicare benefit policy manual* (Pub. 100-02: Ch. 7, Section 30.1.1). Baltimore, MD: Centers for Medicare & Medicaid Services. Retrieved from www.cms.gov/Regulations-and-Guidance/Guidance/Manuals/Downloads/bp102c07.pdf

Centers for Medicare & Medicaid Services. (2003b). *Medicare benefit policy manual* (Pub. 100-02: Ch. 7, Section 30.1.2). Baltimore, MD: Centers for Medicare & Medicaid Services. Retrieved from www.cms.gov/Regulations-and-Guidance/Guidance/Manuals/Downloads/bp102c07.pdf

Centers for Medicare & Medicaid Services. (2011). *Medicare benefit policy manual* (Pub. 100-02: Ch. 7, Section 40.2.1). Baltimore, MD: Centers for Medicare & Medicaid Services. Retrieved from www.cms.gov/Regulations-and-Guidance/Guidance/Manuals/Downloads/bp102c07.pdf

Centers for Medicare & Medicaid Services. (2012). *Outcome and assessment information set: OASIS-C guidance manual* (Chapter 1). Baltimore, MD: Centers for Medicare & Medicaid Services. Retrieved from www.cms.gov/Medicare/Quality-Initiatives-Patient-Assessment-Instruments/HomeHealthQualityInits/HHQIOASISUserManual.html

Centers for Medicare & Medicaid Services. (2013). *Medicare hospice data.* Retrieved from www.cms.gov/Medicare/Medicare-Fee-for-Service-Payment/Hospice/Medicare_Hospice_Data.html

Cole, M. B. (2012). *Group dynamics in occupational therapy: The theoretical basis and practice application of group intervention* (4th ed.). Thorofare, NJ: SLACK Incorporated.

Early, M. B. (2009). *Mental health concepts and techniques for the occupational therapy assistant* (4th ed.). Baltimore, MD: Lippincott Williams & Wilkins.

Edwards, S. J., Buckland, D. J., & McCoy-Powlen, J. D. (2002). *Developmental & functional hand grasps.* Thorofare, NJ: SLACK Incorporated.

Fairchild, S. L. (2013). *Pierson and Fairchild's principles & techniques of patient care* (5th ed.). St. Louis, MO: Saunders.

Gallagher, S. (2005). A third-grader with attention deficit hyperactivity disorder. In K. Sladyk & S. E. Ryan (Eds.), *Ryan's occupational therapy assistant: Principles, practice issues, and techniques* (4th ed.) (pp. 184-200). Thorofare, NJ: SLACK Incorporated.

Gately, C. A., & Borcherding, S. (2012). *Documentation manual for occupational therapy: Writing SOAP notes* (3rd ed.). Thorofare, NJ: SLACK Incorporated.

George, A. H. (2013). Infection control and safety issues in the clinic. In H. M. Pendleton, & W. Schultz-Krohn (Eds.), *Pedretti's occupational therapy: Practice skills for physical dysfunction* (7th ed.) (pp. 140-156). St. Louis, MO: Mosby.

Hellen, C. R., & Padilla, R. (2012). Working with elders who have dementia and Alzheimer's disease. In R. L. Padilla, S. Byers-Connon, & H. L. Lohman (Eds.), *Occupational therapy with elders: Strategies for the COTA* (3rd ed.) (pp. 275-289). Maryland Heights, MO: Elsevier Mosby.

Küpper, L. (Ed.). (2012). The basics of early intervention: 9 key definitions in early intervention (Section 3 of Module 1). *Building the legacy for our youngest children with disabilities: A training curriculum on Part C of IDEA 2004.* Washington, DC: National Dissemination Center for Children with Disabilities. Retrieved from http://nichcy.org/laws/idea/legacy/partc/module1

Morreale, M. J., & Borcherding, S. (2013). *The OTA's guide to documentation: Writing SOAP notes* (3rd ed.). Thorofare, NJ: SLACK Incorporated.

Oakes, C. (2010). Safety and support. In K. Sladyk, K. Jacobs, & N. MacRae (Eds.), *Occupational therapy essentials for clinical competence* (pp. 55-64). Thorofare, NJ: SLACK Incorporated.

Pendzick, M. J., & Rockwell, D. L. (2009). Interventions for education. In J. V. DeLany & M. J. Pendzick, *Working with children and adolescents: A guide for the occupational therapy assistant* (pp. 265-289). Upper Saddle River, NJ: Pearson Education.

Pfeiffer, J., & Jones, J. (1977). *Reference guide to handbooks and annuals* (2nd ed.). La Jolla, CA: University Associates.

Ross, M. (1997). *Integrative group therapy: Mobilizing coping abilities with the five-stage group.* Bethesda, MD: American Occupational Therapy Association.

Siegel, J. D., Rhinehart, E., Jackson, M., Chiarello, L., & the Healthcare Infection Control Practices Advisory Committee. (2007). *2007 guideline for isolation precautions: Preventing transmission of infectious agents in healthcare settings.* Retrieved from www.cdc.gov/hicpac/pdf/isolation/Isolation2007.pdf

Steva, B. J. (2010). Interventions in school and work. In K. Sladyk, K. Jacobs, & N. MacRae (Eds.), *Occupational therapy essentials for clinical competence* (pp. 187-198). Thorofare, NJ: SLACK Incorporated.

Tufano, R. (1997). Therapeutic communication. In K. Sladyk (Ed.), *OT student primer: A guide to college success* (pp. 223-240). Thorofare, NJ: SLACK Incorporated.

Tufano, R. (2003). Mental health occupational therapy (Suicidality: section 6-31). In K. Sladyk (Ed.), *OT study cards in a box.* Thorofare, NJ: SLACK Incorporated.

Tufano, R. (2005). Group intervention. In K. Sladyk & S. E. Ryan (Eds.), *Ryan's occupational therapy assistant: Principles, practice issues, and techniques* (4th ed.) (pp. 382-396). Thorofare, NJ: SLACK Incorporated.

U.S. Department of Education. (n.d.). *Building the legacy: IDEA 2004.* Retrieved from http://idea.ed.gov

Chapter 7

Assessing and Documenting Client Function

A client's level of function is determined through various means, such as skilled observation, formal and informal assessments, and interviews with client or family/significant others. The OT is responsible for directing and documenting the initial evaluation and establishing the occupational therapy intervention plan (American Occupational Therapy Association [AOTA], 2009, 2010). The OTA collaborates with the OT to perform select, delegated tasks to help assess and document client function and implement skilled interventions—all in accordance with regulatory guidelines and payer requirements (AOTA, 2009, 2010). During each intervention session, occupational therapy practitioners use clinical judgment to ascertain safety, changes in the client's situation, areas of progress, and specific factors impeding progress. This chapter provides worksheets and learning activities to help you determine and document levels of function accurately, and implement various assessments correctly. Answers to worksheet exercises are provided at the end of the chapter.

Contents

Morreale, M. J.
Developing Clinical Competence: A Workbook for the OTA (pp. 207-237).
© 2015 SLACK Incorporated.

Worksheet 7-1

Determining Assist Levels

Indicate the specific type of cues or level of assistance (i.e., contact guard, moderate, maximum, etc.) you would document for each of the following client scenarios.

1. The client donned socks by herself using a sock aid.

2. After assessing the resident's transfer skills, the OTA determined the resident needs someone next to her for safety in case the resident forgets to lock the wheelchair brakes or moves too quickly.

3. The client needed reminders to look to the left three times during lunch in order to find all the food on the plate.

4. The client required a hydraulic lift to transfer from bed to wheelchair.

5. The resident needed both the OTA and PTA to help him transfer from the wheelchair to the mat, but he was able to bear some weight on his weak leg.

6. During a toothbrushing task, the client could not put the paste on the brush, manipulate or hold the brush; but she did open her mouth, rinse, and spit on command.

7. The OTA noted that after the containers are opened and food is cut, the resident can feed herself.

8. The student zippered her jacket by herself and the OTA told her she did a good job.

Worksheet 7-1 (continued)

Determining Assist Levels

9. The OTA put the crayon in the child's weak hand, helped him hold it, and guided the child's arm so the child could draw a circle.

10. The OTA let the client know that the lunch tray was in her room so the client returned to her room and fed herself.

11. When donning his shirt, the client needed a little help to bring the shirt around his back and line up the first button.

12. During craft group, because sharp objects were present, the OTA sat next to the client who is suicidal.

13. During recess, the OTA looked out the window periodically to monitor and help ensure the child was playing cooperatively with the other children on the playground.

14. While the client was cooking at the stove, the OTA put an arm lightly around the client's back in case the client became unsteady.

15. The client who has chronic obstructive pulmonary disease (COPD) unloaded the dishwasher, but needed several rest breaks in order to complete the task.

16. The client with left neglect could read the newspaper article only after the OTA put a red line at the left margin.

Worksheet 7-1 (continued)

Determining Assist Levels

17. During mealtime, the OTA had to touch the client's arm a few times to prompt the client to bring food to mouth.

18. The child needed help for about half of the shoe-tying task.

19. The client would only remember to take her medicine when her cell phone timer buzzed.

20. The student demonstrated ability to use her power wheelchair well, so the OTA put a smiley face sticker on the wheelchair.

Worksheet 7-2

Assessing Feeding

Chen, a 75-year-old male from China, sustained a myocardial infarction 4 days ago while visiting his adult children in New York. He remains hospitalized since that time. Yesterday the doctor ordered occupational therapy and Chen was evaluated by the OT. The intervention plan includes goals for increasing Chen's activity tolerance for feeding and grooming while seated in a chair. Today the OTA is working with Chen at breakfast and observes that Chen does not make eye contact, is not picking up the utensils, and is shaking his head "no." What do you think might be a reason for Chen's behavior and refusal to eat? List at least 10 possibilities.

Examples: *Chen may be depressed regarding his recent heart attack.*
Chen may not feel hungry at this time, or might have just eaten something else.

1.

2.

3.

4.

5.

6.

7.

8.

9.

10.

Morreale, M. J. (2015). *Developing clinical competence: A workbook for the OTA.* Thorofare, NJ: SLACK Incorporated.

Learning Activity 7-1: Client Interview

Occupational therapy practitioners gather important information by interviewing clients and family/significant others. The focus of an interview and specific questions asked will vary depending on the client's diagnosis and circumstances, the type of practice area, specific services provided, and priorities for care. Besides carefully considering the client's responses, occupational therapy practitioners use skilled observations to assess the client's mood, demeanor, social interaction skills, cognitive abilities, motor skills, etc. For example, is the client able to maintain attention for the duration of the interview? Does the client make eye contact? Can the client maintain an upright sitting posture? Are tremors or spasticity exhibited? Does the client have difficulty recalling or understanding information?

To practice your interview skills, use the form in Figure 7-1 to interview a family member, classmate, or friend. While this form may help to determine a client's social history, develop an occupational profile, or screen for problem areas, it may need to be adapted for different populations or situations. Additionally, this form does not include all of a client's demographic data or insurance information that might be present on a "real" form. Be sure to explain the purpose of the interview and let the person you are interviewing know he or she can choose not to answer any of the questions. It is also important to keep the information confidential, so do not use the person's real name or date of birth on the form. Of course, for an actual client, identifying information would always be included and the occupational therapy practitioner would use therapeutic communication techniques to probe further if the client was not forthcoming or if particular concerns were noted. Review Chapter 1 for tips regarding active listening and asking open versus closed questions.

Following the interview, elicit feedback about your performance from the person you interviewed. For example, did you speak too quickly or use too much technical jargon? Did you ask questions clearly, confidently, and concisely? Did the interview "flow"? Did the person feel that you appeared interested in his or her responses? Did you spend too much time looking at the form and writing rather than focusing directly on the person? Reflect on any difficulties you may have encountered during this experience. Determine what you might have done better or how you could have worded your questions differently. It is also useful to practice interviewing people from different age groups (e.g., a 10 year old and an 80 year old) to compare and contrast factors, such as amount of time required, style of questioning, demeanor of the people being interviewed, their life views, and types of responses.

Feedback elicited:

Difficulties encountered:

Changes needed:

Client Interview Form

Client name: _____   Date: _____
Date of birth: _____   Age: _____
Gender: _____

Diagnosis/medical concerns: _____
_____

Marital status: ☐ Married   ☐ Widowed   ☐ Divorced   ☐ Single   ☐ Domestic partnership
☐ Other_____

Emergency contact: _____
Contact phone number: _____
Relationship to client: _____

Cultural Considerations: _____

Communication: ☐ Intact   ☐ Impaired   ☐ Hard of hearing   ☐ Hearing aid   ☐ Aphasia
☐ Other_____

Level of Education Completed: _____
Special training/skills: _____
Desired skills or education: _____

Work: Type of occupation _____
☐ Presently working   ☐ Works full-time   ☐ Works part-time   ☐ Works from home
☐ Works occasionally   ☐ Retired   ☐ Never worked   ☐ Volunteers _____
What does client like/dislike about present work? _____

Living Situation:
☐ Owns home   ☐ Condo/co-op   ☐ Apartment   ☐ Relative's home   ☐ Assisted living facility
☐ Institution   ☐ Rents a room   ☐ Other _____
Children: ☐ Yes   ☐ No _____
Lives with others: ☐ Yes   ☐ No _____
Stairs/architectural barriers: _____
Pets: ☐ Yes   ☐ No _____

Emergency Preparedness:
☐ Smoke alarm   ☐ CO_2 detector   ☐ Flashlight/batteries   ☐ Fire extinguisher
☐ Personal emergency response system/panic button   ☐ Portable/cell phone   ☐ Bottled water
☐ Nonperishable food and manual can opener

BADL/IADL:
Daily living skills that client needs help with: _____
_____

Dietary considerations: _____

Functional Mobility: Assistance needed ☐ Yes   ☐ No
☐ No devices used   ☐ Cane   ☐ Quad cane   ☐ Walker   ☐ Rollator   ☐ Crutches
☐ Manual wheelchair   ☐ Power wheelchair   ☐ Power mobility scooter   ☐ Other _____

Figure 7-1A. Client interview form (page 1).

Client Interview Form (continued)

Community Mobility: Transportation adequate for needs: ☐ Yes   ☐ No
    ☐ Drives own car   ☐ Relative drives   ☐ Friend drives   ☐ Walks   ☐ Uses a taxi   ☐ Bus   ☐ Train
    ☐ County/town transit for elderly/disabled

Rest and Sleep:
Reported stress level (0 to 10 scale) _____
Hours of sleep per night?_____   Takes naps? _____
Sleep interrupted by: ☐ Pain   ☐ Bathroom needs   ☐ Caregiver responsibilities   ☐ Anxiety   ☐ Noise
    ☐ Other_____

Play/Leisure:
List three favorite activities and frequency:
1. _____
2. _____
3. _____
Hobbies/special interests or talents: _____
Hours per day watching TV:_____
Does client read: ☐ Books   ☐ Newspapers   ☐ Magazines
Amount and type of daily/weekly exercise: _____

Habits Impacting Health:
Tobacco use: _____   Alcohol use: _____
Other: _____

Computer Skills:
    ☐ Excellent   ☐ Good   ☐ Fair   ☐ Poor   ☐ Do not use
Hours per day using computer: ☐ Work_____   ☐ Leisure _____
Computer or leisure skills desired: _____

Social Participation:
Clubs, groups, religious organizations: _____

Easily engages in activities: ☐ Yes   ☐ No
Satisfied with amount of friends: ☐ Yes   ☐ No
Prefers: ☐ Individual activities   ☐ Group activities   ☐ Activities at home   ☐ Activities in community
Barriers to leisure or social participation: _____

Personal Goal: _____
_____
_____

OT/OTA signature:_____

Figure 7-1B. Client interview form (page 2).

Worksheet 7-3

Assessing Client Factors

1. The OT asked an OTA to use a visual analog scale with a particular client. This type of scale is used to measure which of the following?

   A. Weight

   B. Oxygen level

   C. Visual acuity

   D. Pain

2. The handle of a Jamar hydraulic dynamometer can be adjusted to how many different grip positions?

   A. 3

   B. 4

   C. 5

   D. 6

3. When using a Jamar hydraulic dynamometer, the OTA should place the client's upper extremity in which of the following positions?

   A. 90 degrees shoulder flexion, adduction, 90 degrees elbow flexion, forearm in neutral position

   B. 0 degrees shoulder flexion, adduction, 90 degrees elbow flexion, forearm in neutral position

   C. 90 degrees shoulder flexion, adduction, 90 degrees elbow flexion, supination

   D. 0 degrees shoulder flexion, 90 degrees abduction, 90 degrees elbow extension, forearm in neutral position

4. When using a manual sphygmomanometer with a client, an OTA notices it is not inflating when the device is initially squeezed. Which of the following primary actions should the OTA take?

   A. Plug it into a different electrical outlet

   B. Turn the valve in the opposite direction

   C. Change the handle position

   D. Reset the device to zero

5. When using a hand-held pinch meter to test lateral pinch, the OTA should place the client's upper extremity in which of the following positions?

   A. 90 degrees shoulder flexion, adduction, 90 degrees elbow flexion, full pronation

   B. 90 degrees shoulder flexion, adduction, 90 degrees elbow flexion, forearm in neutral position

   C. 0 degrees shoulder flexion, adduction, 90 degrees elbow flexion, forearm in neutral position

   D. 0 degrees shoulder flexion, adduction, 90 degrees elbow flexion, full supination

6. To test a client's pinch strength, an OTA is using a hand-held pinch meter with a manual reset knob. The OTA determines that the pinch meter needle is already set at zero. When the client squeezes the device, the OTA observes that the needle does not move from the zero position to register pinch strength like the device did earlier in the day. This is the only pinch meter in the clinic. What is the primary action the OTA should take?

   A. Turn the pinch meter over and have the client squeeze the device again

   B. Turn the pinch meter knob the opposite way and have the client squeeze the device again

   C. Notify the OT that the device is broken

   D. Contact the facility maintenance/engineering department to ascertain if the device can be fixed

Morreale, M. J. (2015). *Developing clinical competence: A workbook for the OTA*. Thorofare, NJ: SLACK Incorporated.

Worksheet 7-3 (continued)

Assessing Client Factors

7. When using a volumeter to assess edema, the client should immerse the upper extremity until the plastic stop is between which two digits?

    A. Thumb and index

    B. Ring and small

    C. Index and long

    D. Long and ring

8. During an initial evaluation, the OT assessed a client's right hand edema using a volumeter containing tap water. The OT documented the results as 550 mL. One week later the OTA retested the client's same hand and documented the results as 520 mL. However, as there was a problem with the clinic's water supply at that time, the OTA used bottled water to fill the volumeter. The change from 550 to 520 mL is most likely due to:

    A. Decreased edema

    B. Increased edema

    C. OTA tester error

    D. OTA using bottled water rather than tap water

9. A client sustained a dislocation injury to his right index finger PIP joint. An OTA is taking circumferential measurements of the index finger PIP joint and documents the joint measurement as 6.2 cm. A week earlier the same joint measured 5.7 cm. The client's left index finger PIP joint has a measurement of 5.4 cm. As a result, the OTA should document that the client's right PIP joint demonstrates:

    A. Decreased range of motion (ROM)

    B. Decreased edema

    C. Increased edema

    D. An infection

10. An OTA is working with a client diagnosed with COPD who receives oxygen through a nasal cannula. As the client has been exhibiting dyspnea upon exertion, the OT asked the OTA to assess and document vital signs during the client's self-care routine today. The OTA should interpret this as taking measurements for all of the following except:

    A. Oxygen saturation levels

    B. Heart rate

    C. Systolic pressure

    D. Body temperature

Learning Activity 7-2: Evidence-Based Practice—Grip Strength

With a partner, use a dynamometer that has adjustable grip positions, such as a Jamar hydraulic dynamometer. The person being tested should squeeze the dynamometer with the device set at each of the adjustable handle positions. Note grip scores in order, beginning from the narrowest grip position and progressing to the widest handle position. The device should be reset to zero after each squeeze and the person being tested should exert maximum effort for each trial. Plot the measurements on a graph and connect the dots.

1. _____ lbs.

2. _____ lbs.

3. _____ lbs.

4. _____ lbs.

5. _____ lbs.

Measure grip strength again with the dynamometer set at each of the handle positions, resetting to zero after each squeeze. However, this time the person being tested should give less than maximal effort to misrepresent actual strength (as a malingering client might do to avoid showing progress). Note grip scores in order, beginning from the narrowest grip position and progressing to the widest handle position. Plot the measurements on a graph and connect the dots.

1. _____ lbs.

2. _____ lbs.

3. _____ lbs.

4. _____ lbs.

5. _____ lbs.

Now compare the two graphs. Are they similar or different in terms of shapes or slopes? Find five evidence-based articles to determine if graphing the five grip positions is clinically valid when attempting to determine if a client is actually exerting maximum effort or not.

Worksheet 7-4

Assessing Additional Client Factors

1. An OTA is assessing static two-point discrimination for a client who has undergone surgery for a digital nerve repair to his right index finger. When using a Disc-Criminator or aesthesiometer on the fingertip, which of the following measurements would be considered in the normal range?

    A. 1 cm

    B. 5 cm

    C. 5 mm

    D. 8 mm

2. How much pressure should the OTA apply when administering a static two-point discrimination test?

    A. Until the filament begins to bend

    B. 5 mm of pressure

    C. Until the client is able to feel the stimulus

    D. Until the skin blanches

3. An OTA is using Semmes-Weinstein monofilaments to assess a client's sensation. The progression of colors indicating sensation level in order from better to worse is:

    A. Green, blue, purple, red

    B. Green, yellow, red, blue

    C. Blue, green, purple, red

    D. Blue, purple, red, black

4. A pulse oximeter is used in health care to assess which of the following?

    A. Heart rate

    B. Blood pressure

    C. Body mass

    D. Blood oxygen saturation levels

5. An OTA is assessing a client's right upper extremity passive range of motion (PROM). Which of the following observations noted by the OTA would indicate an abnormal end feel?

    A. Shoulder external rotation: Capsular stretch

    B. Wrist flexion: Hard

    C. Elbow flexion: Soft

    D. Elbow extension: Hard

6. An OTA is assessing a client's right upper extremity PROM. Which of the following observations noted by the OTA would indicate a normal end feel?

    A. Shoulder flexion: Springy block

    B. Shoulder abduction: Capsular stretch

    C. Thumb MP flexion: Hard

    D. Elbow extension: Soft

Worksheet 7-4 (continued)

Assessing Additional Client Factors

7. An outpatient client has a diagnosis of adhesive capsulitis. An OTA is assessing the client's active range of motion (AROM) for shoulder flexion. The OTA observes that when the client raises her affected arm, the client elevates her right scapula excessively. Which of the following is least appropriate for the OTA do?

   A. Ask client to perform active shoulder flexion again but tell her to "relax the shoulder"

   B. Document that the client has poor motor planning

   C. Have client perform AROM in front of a mirror

   D. Provide a tactile cue

8. The OT asked an OTA to assess AROM for a client who has cognitive deficits. When the OTA verbally asks the client to follow various upper extremity commands (i.e., "lift your arm up over your head"), the OTA observes that the client is attending but is not performing the motions correctly. What primary action should the OTA take?

   A. Write down simple instructions for these motions

   B. Document that the client is noncompliant

   C. Speak in a louder voice

   D. Demonstrate the active motions

9. An OTA needs to assess sitting balance for a male client who sustained a cerebrovascular accident. Of the following choices, which is the most useful method for the OTA to assess dynamic sitting balance?

   A. Client sitting on edge of bed and remaining stationary with arms folded in lap

   B. Client positioned in Fowler position in bed while self-feeding

   C. Client sitting on the mat and reaching for items on either side

   D. Client sitting in a chair while shaving

10. An OTA is assessing a client's muscle tone for the biceps muscle. Which of the following techniques is most appropriate for the OTA to use to determine muscle tone?

    A. PROM with a quick stretch

    B. PROM with a slow stretch

    C. Active resisted flexion

    D. Active resisted extension

Assessing Muscle Strength

The questions in Worksheets 7-5 and 7-6 assume that the occupational therapy practitioner is performing a *conventional manual muscle test* (MMT) rather than a functional screening to assess the strength of a muscle or muscle groups for particular joint motions. When administering a MMT, the examiner considers the effects of gravity and places the client in test-specific positions (supine, prone, side-lying, sitting, or standing) according to the motions being tested. Depending on a particular client's situation, such as diagnosis, precautions/contraindications, available time, treatment priorities, client mobility, etc., an occupational therapy practitioner might use clinical judgment to modify standard techniques or positions and perform a functional strength test instead. A functional strength test, rather than a standard MMT, might entail having a client remain lying supine in bed or sitting in a wheelchair for all muscle groups being tested. For example, it may be contraindicated or not feasible for a client with a recent total hip replacement or a frail, elderly client to assume a prone position. The methods used should be clearly documented in the client's chart. Use Figure 7-2 to help you with the clinical decision-making process for performing a MMT. It is important to realize that, although most sources are generally consistent in defining the muscle grades of Normal (N), Good (G), Fair (F), Poor (P), Trace (T), and Zero (0), *differences are evident in the definitions of plus (+) and minus (-) muscle grades* (Clarkson, 2013; Flinn, Latham, & Podolski, 2008; Latella & Meriano, 2003; Liska & Gonzelez, 2013; Reese, 2012; Rybski, 2012). The muscle grades used in this section delineate Fair- (F-) as incomplete ROM against gravity (greater than 50%) and Poor+ (P+) as incomplete ROM against gravity (less than 50%) (Clarkson, 2013; Reese, 2012). *Use the grading system and methods that are standard for your facility.*

Some clinical tips when performing a MMT:

- *Always adhere to any precautions and contraindications based on the client's condition and situation.* Not all clients will require a MMT. Not all clients will be able to assume standard test positions safely.

- Use easy-to-understand instructions instead of technical jargon when asking a client to perform a particular active motion. For example, for shoulder flexion, rather than saying, *"Flex your shoulder,"* you might say, *"Lift your arm up over your head"* or *"Reach up to the ceiling."* It is helpful to demonstrate the desired motions.

- An easier way to remember and visualize proper client position is to consider that *motions against gravity move upward toward the ceiling* (i.e., flexion and abduction while seated or standing, horizontal adduction in supine) and the positions *minimizing the effects of gravity allow for motions to be performed parallel to the floor* (i.e., scapula elevation while prone, horizontal abduction while seated, shoulder flexion while side-lying).

- If you observe that the client does not exhibit full AROM, do not automatically assume that weakness or joint problems exist. If you simply provide an additional verbal cue, such as, *"Can you lift your arm up any higher than that?"* or *"Can you turn your hand over any further?"* the client will often exhibit more complete motion.

- A main defining factor in MMT decision making, a baseline, is determining if the client can perform full *available* AROM against gravity (at least a muscle grade of Fair). *If the client is able to do this,* resistance is applied and the resulting muscle grade can then only be: Fair, Fair+, Good, or Normal. (Some facilities also use G+ and G-). If the client does not meet that baseline, there are two options: (1) the client has already demonstrated the criteria for F- or P+ (depending on amount of motion exhibited) and the test is complete, or (2) based on the criteria, the client must be positioned in a gravity reduced position to determine a muscle grade of Poor, Trace, or Zero.

- As means to help with remembering, the author's students have dubbed the muscle grade of F+ as "shake and break," meaning that the muscle can sustain a minimal amount of resistance, but struggles (shakes) with any greater resistance and lowers downward (breaks).

- A joint limitation or contracture does not necessarily indicate decreased strength. When performing a MMT, if AROM and PROM of a particular joint are equal (client moves through *available* joint range), then resistance should be applied to determine strength (Reese, 2012). For example, a bodybuilder with pectoralis muscle bulk may demonstrate limited ROM for the antagonist of horizontal abduction. However, this is would not necessarily signify that the bodybuilder has decreased muscle strength for horizontal abduction.

Worksheet 7-5

Assessing Muscle Strength

1. An OTA is performing a MMT bedside to determine a client's muscle strength for right shoulder flexion. The client, who is seated at the edge of the bed, is unable to initiate lifting his arm into shoulder flexion but exhibits full PROM. To complete the MMT for shoulder flexion, the OTA should place the client in which of the following positions?

    A. Side-lying in bed

    B. Supine

    C. Prone with arm hanging off side of bed

    D. Not applicable as the test is now complete

2. An athlete with a shoulder condition is receiving outpatient occupational therapy. When performing a MMT for shoulder external rotation, the OTA should initially position the client in which of the following positions?

    A. Sitting in a chair

    B. Side-lying in bed

    C. Supine

    D. Prone

3. When performing a MMT for wrist flexion, on what aspect of the client's extremity should the OTA apply resistance?

    A. Volar forearm

    B. Volar palm

    C. Volar digits

    D. Dorsal hand

4. While performing a MMT on a 35-year-old client who has good balance and mobility, the OTA observes that a client cannot shrug his shoulders while sitting in a chair. For this motion, the next position for the OTA to place the client in is which of the following?

    A. Kneeling on a mat

    B. Sitting on edge of bed

    C. Standing

    D. Prone

5. When assessing muscle strength for wrist extension, a client can perform full AROM with his hand resting sideways on the ulnar side (on a tabletop). However, the client is unable to initiate wrist extension with the palm resting face down on the table. The muscle grade is most likely which of the following?

    A. Fair

    B. Fair-

    C. Poor

    D. Trace

Morreale, M. J. (2015). *Developing clinical competence: A workbook for the OTA.* Thorofare, NJ: SLACK Incorporated.

Worksheet 7-5 (continued)

Assessing Muscle Strength

6. A client can perform full active supination against gravity. What is the next step for the MMT for this motion?

   A. Nothing, as test is completed and muscle grade is fair

   B. Nothing, as test is completed and muscle grade is 5/5

   C. Perform PROM to forearm

   D. Apply resistance

7. A patient with COPD exhibits both AROM and PROM for shoulder flexion as 0 to 100 degrees. The client is unable to sustain any resistance applied to the shoulder flexor muscles. What muscle grade should this be documented as?

   A. Poor

   B. Fair

   C. Poor+

   D. Fair+

8. A client exhibits full passive elbow ROM but can only actively flex his elbow ¾ of the range when seated. What muscle grade should this be documented as?

   A. Fair

   B. Fair+

   C. Fair-

   D. Poor

9. When performing a MMT to test muscle strength for horizontal adduction, the OTA should place the client in which start position?

   A. Supine

   B. Sitting

   C. Side-lying

   D. Prone

10. Which of the following clients is likely the most appropriate to place in the standard MMT initial test position to determine strength for internal rotation?

   A. A 40-year-old carpenter presently in the reconditioning phase of therapy following rotator cuff surgery

   B. A 35-year-old athlete with a shoulder condition who is also 3 weeks status post open heart surgery

   C. A 70-year-old homemaker 3 days status post total hip replacement who requires upper body strengthening for walker use

   D. A 45-year-old female who underwent surgery for a mastectomy 1 week ago

Worksheet 7-6

Assessing Muscle Strength—More Practice

1. An OTA is performing a MMT to test a client's muscle strength for shoulder extension (hyperextension). After completing the initial step, the OTA determines the client must be placed in a gravity-reduced position to complete the test which, for that motion, is which of the following positions?

    A. Sitting

    B. Standing

    C. Side-lying

    D. Prone

2. When performing a MMT to test muscle strength for shoulder abduction, the OTA observes that the client exhibits 100 degrees AROM and 160 degrees PROM. The OTA should determine that the muscle grade is which of the following?

    A. Fair

    B. Fair+

    C. Fair-

    D. Undetermined, need to further test in a gravity-eliminated position

3. A client can fully flex his biceps muscle against gravity. To complete the MMT for the biceps, the OTA should do which of the following?

    A. Nothing, as the test is now complete and muscle grade is 3/5

    B. Nothing, as test is now complete and muscle grade is 5/5

    C. Place client in gravity-minimized position

    D. Apply resistance

4. When performing a MMT to test muscle strength for shoulder internal rotation, the OTA should apply resistance to what aspect of the client's upper extremity?

    A. Distal forearm with client prone

    B. Distal forearm with client supine

    C. Distal forearm with client sitting

    D. Distal humerus with client prone

5. An OTA is performing a MMT to test a client's muscle strength for MP extension. The OTA should place the client's upper extremity in which start position?

    A. Palm resting face down on table

    B. Hand sideways with ulnar side of hand resting on table

    C. Hand sideways with thumb side of hand resting on table

    D. Hand supported on table with palm facing up

Worksheet 7-6 (continued)

Assessing Muscle Strength—More Practice

6. An OTA observes that the client can only touch his thumb to the index and long fingers. Of the following choices, which muscle is most likely affected?

    A. Flexor digitorum profundus

    B. Opponens pollicis

    C. Abductor digiti minimi

    D. Flexor pollicis longus

7. A client is unable to actively flex his MPs to 70 degrees while simultaneously extending his PIPs and DIPs. PROM is within normal limits. Which muscle is most likely affected?

    A. Lumbricals

    B. Extensor carpi radialis

    C. Flexor digitorum superficialis

    D. Flexor digitorum profundus

8. A client is demonstrating difficulty with tendon gliding following a Zone 2 flexor tendon repair. As a result, the OTA should primarily work toward facilitating movement of which of the following muscles?

    A. Opponens pollicis and opponens digiti minimi

    B. Extensor pollicis longus and extensor pollicis brevis

    C. Flexor carpi radialis and flexor carpi ulnaris

    D. Flexor digitorum profundus and flexor digitorum superficialis

9. A client diagnosed with carpal tunnel syndrome is exhibiting weakness of his median innervated intrinsic muscles. Which of the following muscles are included?

    A. Adductor pollicis, flexor pollicis brevis, opponens pollicis

    B. Flexor pollicis brevis, opponens pollicis, abductor pollicis longus

    C. Opponens pollicis, adductor pollicis, abductor pollicis brevis

    D. Flexor pollicis brevis, opponens pollicis, abductor pollicis brevis

10. A client has a diagnosis of low level ulnar nerve lesion. Which of the following observations by an OTA would be consistent with that condition?

    A. Inability to perform palmar abduction

    B. Inability to flex thumb MP

    C. Inability to flex small finger MP

    D. Inability to flex index finger MP

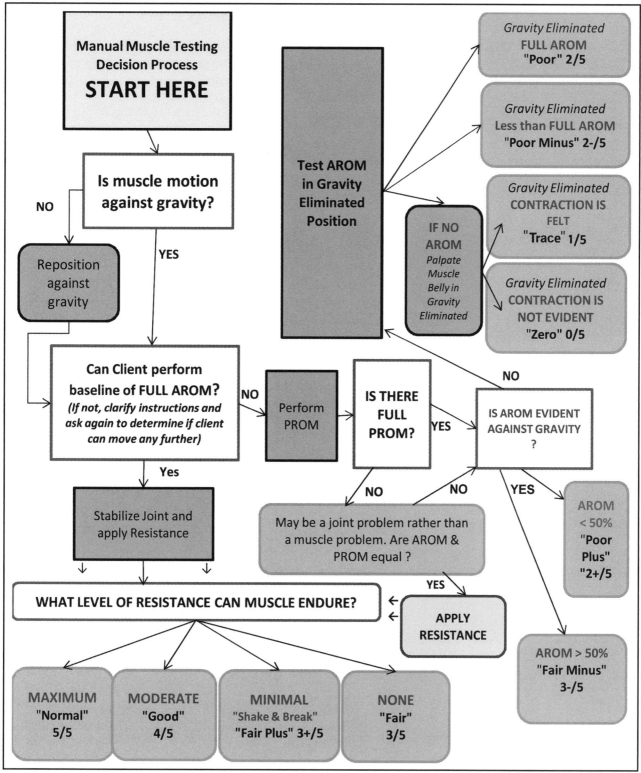

Figure 7-2. Manual muscle test flow chart. (Adapted from Marie Morreale course lecture notes and developed by Elaine Trainor, COTA.)

Learning Activity 7-3: Assessing Pain

As part of a group exercise, participants should create a combined list of situations for which they have experienced (or are currently experiencing) physical pain. Some suggestions are listed as follows, but the group may come up with others. According to each member's comfort level for voluntary disclosure of any personal information, members should describe their personal pain experiences. Consider the particular words needed to specifically describe pain patterns, and to quantify and qualify pain. For example, was the pain throbbing, burning, knife-like, prickly, or achy? Where exactly did the pain occur? Did the pain travel? Was pain constant, intermittent, or perhaps only aggravated by specific motions or activities? What methods, if any, helped to reduce the pain? Compare and contrast the description of pain by several members who have experienced the same conditions. Participants might also discuss the personal effects of pain in regards to their occupational performance. Determine what formal or informal pain scales would be useful to assess pain for each participant's condition or situation.

- Broken bone
- Sprained ankle
- Childbirth
- Kidney stone
- Exercising/working out at the gym
- Back injury/sciatica

- Infection (sinus, ear, wound, urinary tract)
- Headache/migraine
- Pneumonia/pleurisy
- Surgery
- Toothache
- Compressed nerve

Specific Condition	Pain Description	Effect on Occupational Performance	Formal Pain Scales	Informal Pain Scales

Morreale, M. J. (2015). *Developing clinical competence: A workbook for the OTA*. Thorofare, NJ: SLACK Incorporated.

Worksheet 7-7

Behavioral Observation Skills in Mental Health

For each category, list specific behaviors that an occupational therapy practitioner might expect to see in a client who is depressed and how those behaviors might interfere with occupational performance.

1. Intrapersonal factors:

2. Interpersonal behaviors:

3. Task behaviors:

4. Areas of occupation:
    o BADL:

    o Rest and sleep:

    o Leisure:

    o Work/education:

Next, review the following case study. Based on the information provided, look at each of the behaviors you listed and circle only the ones that are actually observed for Laurie while she is on the unit.

Laurie, a 38-year-old bank teller, was admitted to an acute psychiatric unit with a diagnosis of depression. Following her spouse's death from cancer 3 months ago, Laurie states she has stopped attending her weekly college business class and her daily routine of going to the gym. She reports having frequent headaches and muscle tension in her upper back for the past 4 weeks. For the 2 weeks prior to admission, Laurie has stayed in bed all day in her pajamas; missed work; lost weight due to decreased appetite; and has not answered phone calls, text messages, or email. She states that she is "not good enough" to return to work. When asked if she has contacted her college or job to discuss a medical leave, Laurie replied, "Why bother?" She denies suicidal ideation at this time. Laurie does not have any children. She has one sister who lives in the next town, and her parents live in a retirement community 1000 miles away.

Morreale, M. J. (2015). *Developing clinical competence: A workbook for the OTA.* Thorofare, NJ: SLACK Incorporated.

Worksheet 7-8

Improving Observation Skills—Appearance and Hygiene

Clients with conditions such as brain injuries, intellectual disabilities, mental health conditions, or developmental delay require assessment of various factors and skills that reflect mental function, process skills, and ability to interact within social norms. What might you observe and document regarding your client that would indicate a well-groomed appearance versus poor hygiene, health factors, or an unkempt/untidy appearance? In the boxes below, list objective factors pertaining to clothing, skin, face, hair, etc.

Good Hygiene/Well-Groomed Appearance	Poor Hygiene or Health Factors, Unkempt/Untidy Appearance

Morreale, M. J. (2015). *Developing clinical competence: A workbook for the OTA.* Thorofare, NJ: SLACK Incorporated.

Worksheet 7-9

Improving Observation Skills—Mood and Behavior

Clients with conditions such as brain injuries, intellectual disabilities, mental health conditions, or developmental delay require assessment of various factors and skills that reflect mental function, process skills, and ability to interact within social norms. Consider what you might observe and document as indicators of the client's present demeanor, mood, or level of thinking. In the boxes below, list objective factors, such as types of behavior exhibited and statements expressed.

Behavioral Observations (Give Specific Examples of What the Client Actually Did)	Client's Verbalizations (Give Specific Examples of What the Client Actually Said)
Example: Arms crossed in front of chest or not	Example: Client uses courteous words (please, thank you, may I…) or profane words/curses at family, staff, and peers on unit
Example: Attentive or easily distracted (by what internal or external factors)	Example: Verbalizes understanding of deficits or not

Table 7-1 **Levels of Assistance**	

Total assistance (TOT)	Individual requires 100% assistance to safely complete task. Individual does not assist at all.
Maximum assistance (MAX)	Individual requires 75% of physical/cognitive assistance to safely complete task. Individual assists 25%.
Moderate assistance (MOD)	Individual requires 50% of physical/cognitive assistance to safely complete task. Individual assists 50%.
Minimal assistance (MIN)	Individual needs no more than 25% physical/cognitive assistance. Individual assists 75%.
Standby assistance (SBA)	Supervision or standby assistance for safe, effective task performance.
Set-up assistance	Individual requires set-up of necessary items to perform tasks.
Independent (IND)	No assistance or supervision is required. Able to perform independently. Safety is demonstrated during tasks.

Reprinted with permission from Jacobs, K., & Simon, L. (Eds.). (2015). *Quick reference dictionary for occupational therapy* (6th ed.). Thorofare, NJ: SLACK Incorporated.

Answers to Worksheets

Worksheet 7-1: Determining Assist Levels

Resources: Jacobs & Simon, 2015; Logigian, 2005; Morreale & Borcherding, 2013; UB Foundation Activities, Inc. (UBFA, Inc.), 2002

Settings may vary in the specific terminology and criteria used to describe levels of function. Always use the terminology and criteria that are standard for your facility, practice setting, and payer requirements. Examples of commonly used terms and definitions are listed in Table 7-1.

1. <u>Modified independence.</u> The client donned socks by herself using a sock aid.
2. <u>Standby assist.</u> After assessing the resident's transfer skills, the OTA determined the resident needs someone next to her for safety in case the resident forgets to lock the wheelchair brakes or moves too quickly.
3. <u>Three verbal cues or minimal verbal cues.</u> The client needed reminders to look to the left three times during lunch in order to find all the food on the plate.
4. <u>Dependent or total assistance.</u> The client required a hydraulic lift to transfer from bed to wheelchair.
5. <u>Maximum assistance of two persons (max assist X 2).</u> The resident needed both the OTA and PTA to help him transfer from the wheelchair to the mat, but he was able to bear some weight on his weak leg.
6. <u>Maximum assistance.</u> During a toothbrushing task, the client could not put the paste on the brush, manipulate or hold the brush; but she did open her mouth, rinse, and spit on command.
7. <u>Independent with set-up.</u> The OTA noted that after the containers are opened and food is cut, the resident can feed herself.
8. <u>Independent.</u> The student zippered her jacket by herself and the OTA told her she did a good job.
9. <u>Hand-over-hand assistance.</u> The OTA put the crayon in the child's weak hand, helped him hold it, and guided the child's arm so the child could draw a circle.

10. <u>Independent.</u> The OTA let the client know that the lunch tray was in her room so the client returned to her room and fed herself.

11. <u>Minimal assistance.</u> When donning his shirt, the client needed a little help to bring the shirt around his back and line up the first button.

12. <u>Supervision within arm's length or close supervision.</u> During craft group, because sharp objects were present, the OTA sat next to the client who is suicidal.

13. <u>Distant supervision or supervision within line-of-sight.</u> During recess, the OTA looked out the window periodically to monitor and help ensure the child was playing cooperatively with the other children on the playground.

14. <u>Contact guard assistance.</u> While the client was cooking at the stove, the OTA put an arm lightly around the client's back in case the client became unsteady.

15. <u>Modified independence.</u> The client who has COPD unloaded the dishwasher but needed several rest breaks in order to complete the task.

16. <u>Visual cue.</u> The client with left neglect could read the newspaper article only after the OTA put a red line at the left margin.

17. <u>Several tactile cues or minimal physical prompting.</u> During mealtime, the OTA had to touch the client's arm a few times to prompt the client to bring food to mouth.

18. <u>Moderate assistance.</u> The child needed help for about half of the shoe-tying task.

19. <u>Auditory cue.</u> The client would only remember to take her medicine when her cell phone timer buzzed.

20. <u>Independent.</u> The student demonstrated ability to use her power wheelchair well, so the OTA put a smiley face sticker on the wheelchair.

Worksheet 7-2: Assessing Feeding

It is important to look at the client holistically, consider all the possibilities, and determine which of these are applicable to Chen's situation:

1. Chen may be awaiting medical tests for which he is not allowed to eat prior to the test.
2. Chen may not like the food choices, as they may be very different than typical food in China.
3. If ethnic food is available, it may be bland or not appealing due to a possible low-salt or low-fat diet.
4. Chen may normally use chopsticks and may not be comfortable using silverware (Asher, 2006).
5. Food may not conform to the client's values or beliefs, such as religious considerations or if Chen is a vegetarian and meat was served.
6. Chen may be embarrassed to have someone helping him or watching him eat, particularly if the person is a different gender.
7. Chen may have difficulty chewing due to missing teeth or a painful jaw.
8. Chen may have dentures that are not currently in place or are ill-fitting and painful.
9. Chen may have nausea, indigestion, or a stomach ache due to constipation or medication.
10. Chen may be very tired or in pain.
11. Chen may have a poor body image or may have an eating disorder.
12. Chen may have underlying cognitive impairment or perceptual problems.
13. Chen may be waiting for his family to arrive before he eats.

Worksheet 7-3: Assessing Client Factors

1. D. This is a simple and common pain scale (Flinn et al., 2008).
2. C. Lafayette Instrument, 2004.
3. B. Clarkson, 2013; Lafayette Instrument, 2004.
4. B. A sphygmomanometer is a blood pressure device. When using a manual blood pressure device, if the bulb's air valve (knob) is not turned in the proper direction to close it, the cuff will not inflate. This device does not use electricity and automatically starts at zero when the cuff is deflated.
5. C. Clarkson, 2013; Flinn et al., 2008.

6. B. In this instance, the knob was probably turned the wrong way so that the peak-hold needle (which indicates the measurement) is behind, rather than in front of, the gauge needle that is supposed to push it.

7. D. Flinn et al., 2008.

8. A. Bottled versus tap water should not have an effect on test results. Less water was displaced, indicating decreased edema.

9. C. When taking circumferential measurements, an increased number usually indicates increased edema (although girth can also increase due to other factors, such as a nodule, ganglion, cyst, etc.). While the client could be getting an infection, there are no clinical signs indicated for that, such as increased pain, redness, or increased temperature of digit. ROM measurements are not noted in this example.

10. D. The OTA should measure the client's blood pressure, oxygen saturation levels, pulse rate, and note respiration rate/shortness of breath. While it may be appropriate to assess temperature in certain situations, such as for a suspected fever or joint infection, it is not indicated in this situation.

Worksheet 7-4: Assessing Additional Client Factors

1. C. Bentzel, 2008.

2. D. Bentzel, 2008.

3. A. Bentzel, 2008.

4. D.

5. B. Clarkson, 2013.

6. B. Clarkson, 2013.

7. B. The client appears to be compensating for weakness in shoulder flexors rather than demonstrating poor motor planning. The OTA should try methods to minimize muscle substitution.

8. D. Demonstration would help the client to better process the desired motions. Written instructions could be more confusing and, unless the client has hearing impairment or is demonstrating poor attention, a louder voice would not help the situation.

9. C. Of the choices provided, sitting unsupported on a mat and weight shifting to either side would best challenge dynamic sitting balance. However, it would be even more challenging if the client were reaching for objects and weight shifting while seated on edge of bed (which is an unstable surface) rather than a stable mat surface.

10. A. A quick stretch to a muscle is the traditional evaluation to determine if resistance occurs as a response to the movement (Gillen, 2011).

Worksheet 7-5: Assessing Muscle Strength

References: Clarkson, 2013; Reese, 2012

Clinical judgment is needed to determine if modifications are needed for a particular client. These answers are based on standard MMT procedure. As previously noted, *motions against gravity move upward toward the ceiling* (i.e., flexion and abduction while seated/standing, horizontal adduction in supine) and the positions *minimizing the effects of gravity allow for motions to be performed parallel to the floor* (scapula elevation while prone, horizontal abduction while seated, shoulder flexion while side-lying). *Remember, it may not be safe or feasible for some clients to assume a standard test position.*

1. A. The OTA needs to put the client in a gravity-reduced position, which, in this situation, is side-lying. The OTA should support the client's arm or use a powder board.

2. D. The against-gravity start position for external rotation is a prone position. However, this position may be too difficult for elderly clients or contraindicated for some conditions.

3. B. The test begins with client's arm resting on the table with palm facing up. The client flexes the wrist and the OTA applies pressure on the palm in a downward direction.

4. D. A prone position minimizes effects of gravity for scapula elevation. Assuming a prone position may be difficult for elderly clients or contraindicated for some conditions.

5. C. The muscle grade is poor as the client is able to perform the motion in a gravity-reduced plane, but cannot move against gravity.

6. D. The test is not yet complete. The OTA has determined the client demonstrates at least a Fair muscle grade, but needs to apply resistance to complete the MMT.

7. B. The client's present maximum joint range is 100 degrees. While the ROM deficit is documented as a joint contracture, active and passive ranges are equal so the client has at least Fair muscle strength. Resistance is then applied to complete the test, which, in this case, the client cannot sustain so the muscle grade is Fair.

8. C. The client is unable to perform full AROM against gravity, but performs more than 50% of the motion.

9. A. A supine position allows for horizontal adduction to be performed against gravity.

10. A. Resistance is applied to distal forearm with client prone. Resistance and/or a prone position are contraindicated for the other clients due to their medical precautions.

Worksheet 7-6: Assessing Muscle Strength—More Practice

References: Clarkson, 2013; Reese, 2012
Clinical judgment is needed to determine if modifications are needed for a particular client. These answers are based on standard MMT procedure.

1. C. The gravity-reduced position for shoulder extension is side-lying. The OTA should support the client's arm or use a powder board.

2. C. The client demonstrates incomplete AROM against gravity but more than 50% of available joint range.

3. D. The client demonstrates full AROM against gravity, so the next step is to apply resistance.

4. A. The against-gravity start position for internal rotation is a prone position. The position may not be feasible for frail, elderly patients or may be contraindicated for certain conditions (i.e., recent total hip replacement).

5. A. The against-gravity start position for MP extension is with the palm facing down.

6. B. The opponens pollicis allows for thumb opposition.

7. A. The motion is performed using the lumbricals.

8. D. A flexor tendon injury in Zone 2 affects differential tendon gliding of the flexor digitorum profundus and flexor digitorum superficialis. Of course, other muscles and joints may be affected due to complications from the injury and/or surgery and also require intervention.

9. D. The adductor pollicis is ulnar nerve innervated. The abductor pollicis longus is an extrinsic muscle and is not innervated by the median nerve.

10. C. Inability to perform palmar abduction or MP flexion of thumb may indicate median nerve impairment. Inability to flex finger MPs may indicate weakness of the lumbricals, which are innervated by both the median nerve (index and long fingers) and ulnar nerve (ring and small fingers).

Worksheet 7-7: Behavioral Observation Skills in Mental Health

Each client is different, but some suggestions are presented below as possible symptoms of depression that an occupational therapy practitioner might observe. Tufano (2003) urges caution when depressed clients show sudden peacefulness and behavioral changes along with sudden declaration that depression is resolved. This new vigor, for some clients, could be an indicator of suicidality (Tufano, 2003). Giving away of items can also be a warning sign. The items in bold are those that are *actually observed* with Laurie on the unit based on the information provided. She may exhibit other behaviors during her hospitalization or during group activities, but these are not noted in the case study.

1. Intrapersonal factors
   o **Expresses feelings of hopelessness, sadness, depression, or suicidal ideation** (note specific statements); *states "not good enough" to return to work and "why bother?"*
   o **Verbalizes negative attributes about self** (note specific statements); *states "not good enough" to return to work*
   o **Expresses negative outlook regarding future or ability to cope** (note specific statements); *regarding contacting her boss and college, Laurie states, "Why bother?"*
   o Crying exhibited
   o **Somatic complaints**; *reports frequent headaches and muscle tension in her upper back*

- o Inability to identify coping mechanisms for dealing with a depressed mood (i.e., does not identify people client can contact to discuss feelings, expresses unwillingness to exercise/go for a 15-minute walk)
2. Interpersonal behaviors
   - o Lack of eye contact (describe situation)
   - o Flat affect/does not smile
   - o Does not initiate conversation
   - o **Uncommunicative or minimal level of engagement in conversation** (note length and type of responses); *does not answer phone calls or respond to text messages or email*
3. Task behaviors
   - o Refuses or minimally participates in group activities (note how often and for how long)
   - o Poor task initiation
   - o Poor decision making (describe what happens when presented with choosing an activity/craft project or components such as colors or materials)
   - o Does not complete project/gives up
   - o Poor attention to detail/does not recognize or correct errors (describe/give examples)
   - o Low frustration tolerance (describe the situation and behavior)
4. Areas of occupation
   - o BADL
     - ‣ **Change in appetite** (note specific amount eaten and/or types of foods); *Laurie has lost weight prior to admission due to decreased appetite. It is not noted if Laurie's eating patterns have changed since she was admitted.*
     - ‣ **Specific weight loss or gain**; *Laurie has lost weight recently due to decreased appetite although exact amount is not noted. This will need to be monitored on unit.*
     - ‣ **Lacks initiation to get out of bed** (note amount of cueing/assistance needed); *prior to admission Laurie had stayed in bed all day. However, it is not noted if she is continuing this pattern of behavior on the unit.*
     - ‣ **Lacks initiation to get dressed or shower** (note amount of cueing/assistance needed); *prior to admission Laurie had stayed in bed all day in her pajamas. However, it is not noted if she is presently getting dressed on the unit.*
     - ‣ Inattention to grooming and hygiene (describe)
   - o Rest and sleep
     - ‣ Atypical amount of time sleeping or inability to sleep (note sleep patterns)
     - ‣ Reports poor sleep quality
   - o Leisure
     - ‣ **Withdraws from regular leisure routine**; *Laurie reports she has stopped her daily routine of going to the gym.*
     - ‣ Does not express interest in resuming leisure activities
     - ‣ Refuses or demonstrates limited participation in leisure activities on unit (specific tasks, length of time, level of participation)
     - ‣ Expresses unwillingness to resume her exercise regimen or go for a 15-minute walk with staff
   - o Work/education
     - ‣ **Misses work or school**; *Laurie reports she has stopped attending her weekly college business class and for the past 2 weeks has also missed work.*
     - ‣ Expresses lack of desire to return to work and/or school
     - ‣ **Difficulty with initiating contact with employer or teachers for a plan to return to work, complete studies, or arrange for a medical leave**; *states, "Why bother?"*

Worksheet 7-8: Improving Observation Skills—Appearance and Hygiene

A client's personal appearance and hygiene could be an indicator of the client's self-image, mood, health, or cognitive status. *However, the mere presence of any unkempt/untidy factors listed in the answer table does not necessarily correlate to deficits in mental functions or social skills and does not necessarily need to be documented.* For example, a client coming to therapy directly from a landscaping or construction job may be wearing garments with large dirt stains or tears. You might even have once had a piece of spinach inadvertently stuck in your teeth! It is also important not to make value judgments based on one's personal fashion preferences, moral standards, or religious beliefs (Morreale & Borcherding, 2013). The occupational therapy practitioner must distinguish between factors, such as a client who may have a long beard to meet religious requirements versus a client who has suddenly stopped shaving due to depression, defiance against his parents' wishes, or not understanding a job's dress code. If a client arrives with make-up applied only to one side of face or with lipstick circling her nose, clinical reasoning will ascertain if these behaviors are influenced by particular deficits, such as left neglect or perhaps a psychotic episode. As another example, a teenager wearing flannel pajama pants at a coffee shop may consider himself fitting in with peers, whereas an 80-year-old adult would likely consider the teen's fashion choice as inappropriate for outside of the home. However, observations such as a client with disordered clothing, needle track marks, or a skeletal appearance may be quite noteworthy. Clinical judgment is always needed to determine behavior patterns, how your observations may be pertinent or significant to the client's present circumstances, and what should be noted in the client's chart.

Good Hygiene/Well-Groomed Appearance	Poor Hygiene or Health Factors, Unkempt/Untidy Appearance
Clean face and skin, no visible dirt or food particles present	Visible dirt or food on face/skin, presence of soap or make-up residue, strong body odor
Hair clean, combed, neatly styled	Hair greasy, dirty, uncombed, matted, presence of lice
Clean teeth, no food particles noted in mouth	Food particles stuck in teeth; gum disease; missing, discolored, or loose teeth
Clothing without wrinkles, neatly pressed, intact	Clothing wrinkled, torn, number/size of holes, presence of multiple lint balls, or large hanging threads/missing buttons
Clothing clean, without stains	Clothing unclean (i.e., has food, grass, or dirt stains; bugs)
Clothing fits properly	Clothing ill-fitting: described as inability to fasten buttons or zipper due to clothing not fitting, clothing several sizes too big, undergarments visible, skirt dragging on floor, etc.
Buttons lined up properly, fastenings closed, shoelaces tied	Fastenings open or misaligned, shoelaces untied or missing
Clothing right side out	Clothing disordered, inside out, or backward
Hat centered on head, socks pulled up	Hat worn backward or falling off, socks down to ankle
Clothing matches and is complete and appropriate for occasion, weather; attention to detail with accessories	Missing an item, such as a sock or shoe, clothing does not match or is not appropriate for weather or occasion.
Clean shaven, facial hair neatly trimmed	Stubble (i.e., several days facial hair growth), length of beard/mustache, blood present from shaving cuts
Make-up neatly applied	Make-up streaked; lipstick, eye liner, or shadow grossly uneven or beyond typical boundaries
Nails clean, neatly shaped, and polished	Visible dirt beneath nails, length or unevenness of nails, brittleness or fungus present
Smooth, intact skin	Flaky skin, rough/scaly patches, thick callous, open sores, acne, rash, presence of needle track marks, scars from self-mutilation/cutting, nicotine stains
Weight in proportion to height	Weight not in proportion to height (i.e., skeletal, morbidly obese), note specific weight and height
Other:	
Other:	

Worksheet 7-9: Improving Observation Skills—Mood and Behavior

Avoid "judgmental" words when describing relevant client actions objectively, and use clinical reasoning to determine how those observations are pertinent to the client's condition or situation and what is noteworthy to document (Morreale & Borcherding, 2013). For example, instead of saying, "Client is paranoid," a better choice of words might be, "Client is exhibiting suspicious behavior such as disassembling his phone and alarm clock several times daily to check if those items are bugged." Here are some suggestions of what to look out for, although you may come up with others.

Behavioral Observations (Give Specific Examples of What the Client Actually Did)	Client Verbalizations (Give Specific Examples of What the Client Actually Said)
Facial expression (i.e., flat affect or smiling, laughing, frowning, tearful/crying)	Identifies mood, such as feelings/thoughts of persecution, depression, happiness, anger, grief, anxiety, guilt, etc.
Eyes open or closed, level of eye contact, looks away	Positive or negative statements about self regarding appearance, abilities, or how others perceive client
Attentiveness, ability to concentrate, easily startled or distracted	Flight of ideas, confusion, lucidity, logical or illogical statements
Head and trunk upright or shoulders hunched, client stooped over	Changes answers/opinions, vacillates, repetitiveness of answers, or replies without thinking
Personal space boundaries	Specific statements that reflect various defense mechanisms (identify with examples)
Arms/legs crossed or open, leans forward or away	Stated opinion regarding future /outlook, past/present rehabilitation, or potential to change
Affectionate behaviors (hugs, kisses), readily shakes hands, or avoids personal contact	Expresses obsessive thoughts, hallucinations, or delusions
Repetitive behavior/rituals or motor activity (i.e., hand wringing, shaking/trembling, tics, nail-biting, thumb-sucking, rocking, spinning, etc.)	Tone and quality of speech, fluency
Client exhibits behaviors such as hitting, kicking, spitting, or hurting others	Client exhibits profane language, yells, screams, or makes other sounds
Threatening approach (points, jabs, is "in one's face")	Client acknowledges or denies problems or deficits
Pacing, timing, and level of energy exhibited (give examples of sedentary, active, manic, impulsive, cautious, reckless, suspicious behavior, etc.)	Client expresses specific realistic or unrealistic fears/anxieties
Alert, awake, energetic versus groggy, sleepy, listless	Client expresses willingness or unwillingness to change thoughts or behavior
Goal-directed behaviors or agitation, restlessness, wandering aimlessly	Client's stated attitude toward completion of task
Sits alone or engages easily with others,	Verbalizes understanding of deficits or not
Tantrums or other types of acting-out behaviors noted	Length of responses, uncommunicative, rambles, or guarded responses
Handling of objects (rough, destroys or throws items, handles carefully, etc.)	Uses tactful, courteous, respectful words or expresses frustration, is argumentative/tries to pick a fight
Avoids or seeks specific sensory stimulation	Stated sleep patterns or changes
Shares items willingly or not (i.e., sitting space, food, cigarettes, craft materials, books/magazines, tools)	Stated changes in weight (time period)
Other:	Asks staff, family, or peers for help when needed
Other:	

Adapted from Morreale, M. J., & Borcherding, S. (2013). *The OTA's guide to documentation: Writing SOAP notes* (3rd ed.). Thorofare, NJ: SLACK Incorporated.

References

American Occupational Therapy Association. (2009). Guidelines for supervision, roles, and responsibilities during the delivery of occupational therapy services. *American Journal of Occupational Therapy, 63*(6), 797-803. doi: 10.5014/ajot.63.6.797

American Occupational Therapy Association. (2010). Standards of practice for occupational therapy. *American Journal of Occupational Therapy, 64*(6 Suppl.), S106-S111. doi: 10.5014/ajot.2010.64S106

Asher, A. (2006). Asian Americans. In M. Royeen & J. L. Crabtree (Eds.), *Culture in rehabilitation: From competency to proficiency* (pp. 151-180). Upper Saddle River, NJ: Pearson Education, Inc.

Bentzel, K. (2008). Assessing abilities and capacities: Sensation. In M. V. Radomski & C. A. T. Latham (Eds.), *Occupational therapy for physical dysfunction* (6th ed.) (pp. 212-233). Baltimore, MD: Lippincott Williams & Wilkins.

Clarkson, H. M. (2013). *Musculoskeletal assessment: Joint motion and muscle testing* (3rd ed.). Philadelphia, PA: Lippincott Williams & Wilkins.

Flinn, N. A., Latham, C. A. T., & Podolski, C. R. (2008). Assessing abilities and capacities: Range of motion, strength, and endurance. In M. V. Radomski & C. A. T. Latham (Eds.), *Occupational therapy for physical dysfunction* (6th ed.) (pp. 91-185). Baltimore, MD: Lippincott Williams & Wilkins.

Gillen, G. (2011). Upper extremity function and management. In G. Gillen (Ed.), *Stroke rehabilitation: A function-based approach* (3rd ed.) (pp. 218-279). St. Louis, MO: Elsevier Mosby.

Jacobs, K., & Simon, L. (Eds.). (2015). *Quick reference dictionary for occupational therapy* (6th ed.). Thorofare, NJ: SLACK Incorporated.

Lafayette Instrument. (2004). *Jamar Hydrolic Hand Dynamometer user instructions.* Retrieved from www.limef.com/downloads/JAMARHandDynamometer.pdf

Latella, D., & Meriano, C. (2003). *Occupational therapy manual for evaluation of range of motion and muscle strength.* Clifton Park, NY: Delmar Learning.

Liska, C., & Gonzelez, T. R. (2013). Assessment of muscle strength. In M. B. Early (Ed.), *Physical dysfunction practice skills for the occupational therapy assistant* (3rd ed.) (pp. 132-155). St. Louis, MO: Mosby.

Logigian, M. (2005). A businessman with a stroke. In K. Sladyk & S. E. Ryan (Eds.), *Ryan's occupational therapy assistant: Principles, practice issues, and techniques* (4th ed.) (pp. 318-332). Thorofare, NJ: SLACK Incorporated.

Morreale, M. J., & Borcherding, S. (2013). *The OTA's guide to documentation: Writing SOAP notes* (3rd ed.). Thorofare, NJ: SLACK Incorporated.

Reese, N. B. (2012). *Muscle and sensory testing* (3rd ed.). St. Louis, MO: Elsevier Saunders.

Rybski, M. F. (2012). *Kinesiology for occupational therapy* (2nd ed.). Thorofare, NJ: SLACK Incorporated.

Tufano, R. (2003). Mental health occupational therapy (suicidality: section 6-31). In K. Sladyk (Ed.), *OT study cards in a box.* Thorofare, NJ: SLACK Incorporated.

UB Foundation Activities, Inc. (2002). Description of the levels of function and their scores. In *IRF-PAI training manual* (section III-7). Retrieved from www.cms.gov/Medicare/Medicare-Fee-for-Service-Payment/InpatientRehabFacPPS/downloads/irfpai-manualint.pdf

Chapter 8

Incorporating Fundamentals of Care

The worksheets and learning activities presented in this final chapter address a variety of areas applicable to occupational therapy practice, including medical information, grading and adapting, department management, billing and reimbursement, and unusual clinical situations. Answers to worksheet exercises are provided at the end of the chapter.

Contents

Morreale, M. J.
Developing Clinical Competence: A Workbook for the OTA (pp. 239-268).
© 2015 SLACK Incorporated.

Worksheet 8-1

Diseases

List another common name for the conditions listed below.

1. Trisomy 21 _____

2. Complex regional pain syndrome _____

3. Lou Gehrig's disease _____

4. Herpes zoster _____

5. Golfer's elbow _____

6. Degenerative joint disease _____

7. Adhesive capsulitis _____

8. Tennis elbow _____

9. Gamekeeper's thumb _____

10. Epstein-Barr virus _____

11. Ewing sarcoma _____

12. Barlow's syndrome _____

13. Varicella _____

14. Decubitus ulcer _____

15. Hypoglycemia _____

16. Myocardial infarction _____

17. Hypertension _____

18. Hyperemesis _____

19. Distal radius fracture _____

20. Hyperlipidemia _____

Worksheet 8-2

Common Medications

Match each of the conditions in the boxes below to one of the medications listed. Although some medications may be used to treat multiple problems, list each of the conditions below only once.

Multiple sclerosis	Infection	Pain	Angina
Osteoarthritis	Hypertension	Schizophrenia	Diabetes
Osteoporosis	Parkinson's disease	Asthma	Shingles
Atrial fibrillation	Cancer	Depression	Dementia
Iron deficiency	Anxiety	Attention deficit disorder	Seizure

1. Warfarin _____

2. Nitroglycerin _____

3. Naproxen _____

4. Aricept _____

5. Risperdal _____

6. Atenolol _____

7. Diazepam _____

8. Boniva _____

9. Levodopa _____

10. Topamax _____

11. Demerol _____

12. Methotrexate _____

13. Adderall _____

14. Lexapro _____

15. Proventil _____

16. Augmentin _____

17. Avonex _____

18. Acyclovir _____

19. Humulin R _____

20. Slow-FE _____

Worksheet 8-3

Generic Medications

Match the brand name medications in the box below to the generic equivalent listed.

Neurontin	Aleve	Tenormin	Valium
Advil	Xanax	Lipitor	Tylenol
Tums	Coumadin	Cymbalta	Cardizem
Vasotec	Humulin R	Prozac	Klonopin
Prilosec	Ventolin	Vicodin	Paxil

1.   Warfarin _____

2.   Omeprazole_____

3.   Ibuprofen _____

4.   Diazepam _____

5.   Naproxen_____

6.   Hydrocodone bitartrate _____

7.   Albuterol_____

8.   Gabapentin _____

9.   Atorvastatin calcium _____

10. Clonazepam _____

11. Enalapril maleate _____

12. Alprazolam _____

13. Insulin_____

14. Fluoxetine hydrochloride _____

15. Diltiazem _____

16. Acetaminophen_____

17. Paroxetine _____

18. Duloxetine hydrochloride_____

19. Calcium carbonate _____

20. Atenolol_____

Morreale, M. J. (2015). *Developing clinical competence: A workbook for the OTA.* Thorofare, NJ: SLACK Incorporated.

Worksheet 8-4

Occupational Therapy Practice Framework

A person's daily activities can be classified as the various occupations delineated in the *Framework* (American Occupational Therapy Association [AOTA], 2014). However, some activities may not fit neatly into a single *Framework* category, depending on the perspective of the individual or population's interests and needs (AOTA, 2014). For example, making bread may be classified as an IADL (meal preparation), a leisure activity for someone whose hobby is baking, or may be considered social participation or volunteer work if a group is making Challah bread for a religious service or a fundraising event.

Indicate which area(s) of occupation that each of the listed items belong to, according to your personal interests, values, and roles.

Client Activity	BADL	IADL	Play	Leisure	Work	Education	Rest and Sleep	Social Participation
Baking bread								
Cleaning contact lenses								
Taking the train to get to a job								
Donning a splint								
Playing hopscotch with others								
Attending religious services								
Making a collage for an OTA class homework assignment								
Watching TV to fall asleep								
Feeding the household cat or dog								
Listening to music								
Preparing a résumé								
Functional ambulation								
Taking a nap								
Babysitting a younger sibling								
Organizing school papers into folders								
Volunteering at a hospital gift shop								
Attending a bridal shower or bachelor party								
Paying bills								
Getting to next class on time								
Knitting a sweater to wear								
Using contraception								

Worksheet 8-4 (continued)

Occupational Therapy Practice Framework

Client Activity	BADL	IADL	Play	Leisure	Work	Education	Rest and Sleep	Social Participation
Setting an alarm clock								
Reading emails								
Taking vitamins								
Sewing a button back on a shirt								
Planting flowers in the yard								
Writing a performance review for a staff member								
Navigating a wheelchair in the home								
Dressing a doll								
Exercising at the gym								
Calling 911 when smelling smoke								
Eating lunch with colleagues								

Worksheet 8-5

Grading and Adapting—Making Coffee

List ways to grade and adapt the occupation of making coffee by indicating various modifications for the activity demands designated at the top of each column.

Activity Demand: Task Material—Coffee	Activity Demand: Required action of opening coffee container	Activity Demand: Required action of measuring coffee	Activity Demand: Required action of heating the water/brewing coffee
Example: Instant coffee	Example: Can of coffee requiring use of a can opener	Example: Use a measuring spoon	Example: Boil water in teakettle using stove

Morreale, M. J. (2015). *Developing clinical competence: A workbook for the OTA*. Thorofare, NJ: SLACK Incorporated.

Worksheet 8-6

Grading and Adapting—Laundry

List the sequence of steps to wash clothes and various ways to grade and adapt each of those steps.

Sequence of Steps to Perform the Occupation of Laundry	Grade/Adapt Task Methods	Grade/Adapt Task Materials
Example: Carry a laundry basket full of clothes to washer	Example: Place dirty clothes directly in machine when getting changed	Example: Use a rolling laundry cart Use a laundry bag

Morreale, M. J. (2015). *Developing clinical competence: A workbook for the OTA.* Thorofare, NJ: SLACK Incorporated.

Learning Activity 8-1: Preparing Breakfast (Traumatic Brain Injury)

Your client is a 35-year-old female recovering from a traumatic brain injury. She exhibits deficits in organization, problem solving, and safety, but does not have any impairment in range of motion, strength, or endurance.

For the occupation of preparing breakfast, put the following items in order of difficulty from easier to harder for this client scenario. Indicate the activity demands that make each task easier or harder. Compare your answers for this exercise to your answers for Learning Activity 8-2. Is your order of difficulty the same or different?

A. Scrambled eggs and bacon

B. Frozen breakfast sandwich

C. Cereal and milk

D. Smoothie (made from scratch)

E. Hard-boiled eggs

F. Frozen waffles

G. Toast

H. Pancakes (using a mix)

I. Yogurt

J. Fresh fruit salad (apple, grapes, melon)

List Tasks in Order of Difficulty From Easiest to Hardest	Rationale
1.	
2.	
3.	
4.	
5.	
6.	
7.	
8.	
9.	
10.	

Learning Activity 8-2: Preparing Breakfast (Rheumatoid Arthritis)

Your client is a 65-year-old female with severe rheumatoid arthritis. She has multiple joint contractures in both hands and is unable to make a full fist or perform tip pinch.

For the occupation of preparing breakfast, put the following items in order of difficulty from easier to harder for this client scenario. Indicate the activity demands that make each task easier or harder. Compare your answers for this exercise to your answers for Learning Activity 8-1. Is your order of difficulty the same or different?

- A. Scrambled eggs and bacon
- B. Frozen breakfast sandwich
- C. Cereal and milk
- D. Smoothie (made from scratch)
- E. Hard-boiled eggs
- F. Frozen waffles
- G. Toast
- H. Pancakes (using a mix)
- I. Yogurt
- J. Fresh fruit salad (apple, grapes, melon)

List Tasks in Order of Difficulty From Easiest to Hardest	Rationale
1.	
2.	
3.	
4.	
5.	
6.	
7.	
8.	
9.	
10.	

Worksheet 8-7

Billing and Reimbursement

1. A 75-year-old client who receives outpatient rehabilitation has Medicare B as his primary health insurance. The OTA and PTA work together with the client for 30 minutes to instruct the client in safe transfers. The PT plans to bill Medicare for two units of therapy. How many units should the OTA bill Medicare for this co-treatment?

   A. 0

   B. 1

   C. 2

   D. 3

2. A client in a skilled nursing facility has Medicare B as his primary health insurance. An OTA works with the client in occupational therapy, providing 20 minutes of ADL training. How many units can the OTA bill Medicare for the therapy provided?

   A. 1

   B. 2

   C. 5

   D. 20

3. An OTA is working in an acute care hospital with a 65-year-old inpatient who is a retired businessman. Of the following choices, the third-party payer for the client's health care is most likely which of the following?

   A. TRICARE

   B. Medicare Part A

   C. Medicare Part B

   D. Medicare Part D

4. An OTA is working on an acute psychiatric unit with a 72-year-old client who is a retired factory worker. The client has Medicare as his primary health insurance. The facility will most likely be reimbursed through which of the following?

   A. Medicare Part A Prospective Payment System

   B. Medicare Part B Physician Fee Schedule

   C. Medicare Part D Rehabilitation Fee Schedule

   D. Medicare Part B Therapy Cap

5. An OTA is working in an outpatient clinic. A client in occupational therapy is 45 years old and has private insurance that pays 80% of health care costs after a $150 deductible is met. The client's occupational therapy evaluation last week cost $100 and today is the client's first treatment session which costs $70. The client has not had any other health services this calendar year. How much money out-of-pocket will the client have to pay for today's session?

   A. $20

   B. $54

   C. $56

   D. $70

Worksheet 8-7 (continued)

Billing and Reimbursement

6. Which of the following is a mandatory insurance that businesses pay to cover the health costs of workers who are injured on the job?

   A. TRICARE

   B. Unemployment Insurance

   C. Medicare Part C

   D. Workers' Compensation

7. Which of the following does not meet the Medicare criteria to be classified as durable medical equipment?

   A. Wheelchair

   B. Commode

   C. Tub seat

   D. Quad cane

8. A 14-month-old child with a developmental delay would most likely receive occupational therapy services resulting from which legislation?

   A. OBRA

   B. IDEA Part B

   C. IDEA Part C

   D. HIPAA

9. Which of the following choices is most likely the third-party payer for health care for an unmarried 28-year-old female who has been unemployed for 12 months, is pregnant, and has no assets?

   A. Unemployment insurance

   B. Supplemental Security Insurance

   C. Workers' Compensation

   D. Medicaid

10. An OTA provides 30 minutes of therapy to a 50-year-old outpatient client who is recovering from a shoulder fracture. The OTA is unsure as to what the proper billing codes are for therapeutic exercise and ADL retraining. Which of the following would be the most useful resource?

    A. International Classification of Diseases manual

    B. Medicare Benefit Policy Manual

    C. Current Procedural Terminology manual

    D. Minimum Data Set

Learning Activity 8-3: Billing Codes

Current Procedural Terminology (CPT) are standard billing codes that are part of the Healthcare Common Procedure Coding System and are used to bill insurance companies for individual skilled health services, such as outpatient occupational therapy (Centers for Medicare & Medicaid Services [CMS], 2011). Billing for some therapy procedures is based on units of time (in 15-minute increments). Other procedures are considered untimed and billed only one unit regardless of the time provided for that service (CMS, 2011). Use a CPT manual (found at a library, fieldwork site, or online) to find the correct billing codes for the following occupational therapy interventions. Determine what general intervention category the specific tasks come under, if it is considered a timed service, and if constant attendance or one-on-one care by the occupational therapy practitioner is required or not. An example is provided.

OT Intervention Implemented	Billing Category	Is This Intervention Considered Timed or Untimed?	Is This Intervention Considered as Only a Supervised Modality or Is It Classified as Requiring Constant Attendance or One-on-One With an OT Practitioner?	CPT Billing Code
Example: *Upper extremity coordination exercises*	*Neuromuscular reeducation*	*Timed*	*One-on-one intervention*	*97112*
Teaching use of a buttonhook				
Measuring a client for a wheelchair				
Instruction and practice using worksheets to improve sequencing and problem solving				
Using a hot pack				
Checking and modifying a splint				
Assessing upper extremity strength				
Teaching compensatory techniques for cooking				
Educating a client in sliding board transfers				
Hand strengthening using a hand gripper and therapy putty				
Assessing a client's home for safety				
Teaching coping strategies to a client who abuses alcohol				
Teaching a client how to propel and use a wheelchair				
Paraffin treatment				

Morreale, M. J. (2015). *Developing clinical competence: A workbook for the OTA.* Thorofare, NJ: SLACK Incorporated.

Learning Activity 8-4: Diagnosis Codes

The World Health Organization maintains a standard, universal listing of codes for diseases and conditions, called the International Classification of Diseases (ICD), which is periodically revised (2013). The United States will be shifting from using version ICD-9 to the use of ICD-10, effective October 1, 2015, as mandated by the U.S. Department of Health and Human Services (American Academy of Professional Coders, 2014). For the conditions listed below, use a current ICD manual to look up each of the diagnosis codes. Realize that the condition may be listed as a synonym in the ICD manual.

1. Parkinson's disease _____

2. A cut to the index finger _____

3. Marfan syndrome _____

4. Middle cerebral artery subarachnoid hemorrhage _____

5. Cubital tunnel syndrome _____

6. Down syndrome _____

7. Failure to thrive (child) _____

8. Schizophrenia _____

9. Glaucoma _____

10. Ulnar shaft open fracture _____

Worksheet 8-8

Department Management

Occupational therapy practitioners planning to establish a private practice therapy program or clinic must first create a sound business plan, carefully considering factors such as the potential client base, likely funding sources (i.e., Medicare, Workers' Compensation, early intervention, private insurance, client self-pay, etc.), and available budget. Reimbursement from third-party payers is normally contingent on meeting very strict criteria in order to be able to bill that insurer for therapy, such as becoming a Medicare-certified agency or being part of an insurer network. In addition, there are many legal and logistical factors involved with owning or managing a program or clinic. As a creative exercise, imagine that you and an OT have decided to open up a private outpatient therapy clinic together. Consider the following factors in regard to this endeavor.

1. *Vision:* Determine what your vision is for this new program and decide on a name for the program or facility. Consider the geographic area (i.e., county, entire state, multiple states) and client population that the clinic will likely serve (i.e., infants, school-age children, adults, elderly). Decide on the specific types of services that will be offered (i.e., health and wellness, adult rehabilitation, sensory integration, driver rehabilitation, low vision, hand therapy). Looking toward the future, consider if your plans would include eventually expanding the clinic or establishing other sites.

    Vision for private practice:

    A. Name of facility: _____

    B. Geographic area: _____

    C. Type of practice area: _____

    D. Population served:_____

    E. Services offered: _____

    F. Likely funding sources:_____

    G. Future plans: _____

2. *Space:* Besides the cost, determine at least 10 criteria to consider when looking for a suitable space to rent or buy:

    A. _____

    B. _____

    C. _____

    D. _____

    E. _____

    F. _____

    G. _____

    H. _____

    I. _____

    J. _____

3. *Equipment and supplies:* Assume you have rented empty space and now need to purchase all the equipment and supplies for this clinic. Brainstorm a list of items that will be needed. Prioritize the items into three categories: Items that are essential for day 1, items that are needed but do not have to be purchased immediately, and a "wish-list" of items that will be purchased as revenue increases. Do not include professional expenses such as insurance, building permits, and licensing fees in this list.

Morreale, M. J. (2015). *Developing clinical competence: A workbook for the OTA.* Thorofare, NJ: SLACK Incorporated.

Worksheet 8-8 (continued)

Department Management

Category	Essential Items	Needed but Can Be Deferred	Wish List
Safety			
Office furniture			
Office equipment			
Office supplies			
Evaluation tools			
General supplies			
Exercise equipment			
ADL equipment			
Adaptive equipment			
Physical agent modalities			
Splinting supplies			
Other:			
Other:			

4. *Possible staff and professional services needed:* Besides possibly hiring other occupational therapy practitioners, list at least eight other disciplines or services you may need to pay for when starting or owning a private practice. Do not include other rehabilitation disciplines, such as physical or speech therapy.

A. _____

B. _____

C. _____

D. _____

E. _____

F. _____

G. _____

H. _____

Morreale, M. J. (2015). *Developing clinical competence: A workbook for the OTA.* Thorofare, NJ: SLACK Incorporated.

Worksheet 8-9

Budget

Indicate if the following statements are true or false.

1. T ____   F ____   A fiscal year goes from January 1 to December 31.

2. T ____   F ____   An example of an occupational therapy capital budget expenditure is a tub seat.

3. T ____   F ____   Revenue equals total income minus expenses.

4. T ____   F ____   An example of a fixed cost is rent.

5. T ____   F ____   Accounts receivable includes the money due from an insurance company.

6. T ____   F ____   An example of variable expenses are office supplies.

7. T ____   F ____   Nonprofit means that the organization does not meet its expenses.

8. T ____   F ____   Total costs subtracted from revenue equals profits.

9. T ____   F ____   An occupational therapy department budget always contains money for staff to attend continuing education seminars to maintain NBCOT certification.

10. T ____   F ____   Costs for items ordered but not paid for are considered accounts payable.

11. T ____   F ____   Bandages, lotions, and paraffin are considered direct use supplies.

12. T ____   F ____   Cash flow consists of pending money due from third-party payers.

13. T ____   F ____   Expenses that are fixed, such as salaries and equipment leases, are called overhead.

14. T ____   F ____   Productivity refers to the amount of billable services that an individual provides.

15. T ____   F ____   A piece of capital equipment that is depreciating is considered an asset.

© SLACK Incorporated, 2015.
Morreale, M. J. (2015). *Developing clinical competence: A workbook for the OTA*. Thorofare, NJ: SLACK Incorporated.

Learning Activity 8-5: Mission Statements

Choose two health-related facilities in your community, such as a hospital, doctors' group, or outpatient rehabilitation clinic. One facility should be classified as a not-for-profit organization and the other a for-profit organization. Using the company websites, locate the mission statements for both facilities and compare and contrast them.

	Not-for-Profit Health Facility	For-Profit Health Facility
Name of facility/organization		
Is this facility part of a larger network or organization? If so, describe.		
Overall philosophy (i.e., religious, philanthropic, social justice)		
Population served (geographic area and/or types of diagnoses)		
List three primary services provided to the community it serves	1. 2. 3.	1. 2. 3.
List five words from the mission statement that best convey the values of the organization	1. 2. 3. 4. 5.	1. 2. 3. 4. 5.
Stated vision for the future		

Morreale, M. J. (2015). *Developing clinical competence: A workbook for the OTA.* Thorofare, NJ: SLACK Incorporated.

Handling Situations Appropriately

An OTA must perform professional duties competently, such as selecting and implementing appropriate interventions, documenting client care, and completing departmental tasks within acceptable time frames. In addition, an OTA must "expect the unexpected" and be prepared to handle unpredictable situations that may occur during the course of the workday. It is essential that an OTA demonstrate good clinical judgment and respond swiftly and appropriately when faced with emergency situations, difficult client behaviors, safety issues, unusual occurrences, and ethical concerns (AOTA, 2010a, 2010b). As you complete Learning Activities 8-6 and 8-7, consider the suggestions in Table 8-1 for managing atypical (i.e., difficult or unusual) situations.

Table 8-1
Handling Situations Appropriately

- Remain calm
- Exercise prudence
- Obtain help as needed
- Use good clinical reasoning
- Demonstrate professionalism and sensitivity
- Incorporate therapeutic use of self
- Maintain client dignity
- Do what is in the best interest of the client
- Make safety a priority
- Know relevant emergency procedures and undergo training for first aid/CPR
- Utilize proper infection control techniques
- Understand liability issues
- Keep current with legislation influencing occupational therapy practice
- Complete documentation requirements
- Adhere to facility policies and procedures
- Follow-up as needed
- Notify your supervisor and appropriate others according to facility policy and relevant laws
- Implement preventative measures
- Learn from the experience
- Maintain healthy habits and manage your own stress level for optimal work performance

Learning Activity 8-6: Handling Situations Appropriately

Indicate how you would respond appropriately with *professionalism and sensitivity* to the following actual clinical situations that various occupational therapy practitioners have encountered (identifying details have been changed). Consider what you would say to the clients, the immediate action you would take, and any follow-up that may be required.

1. Marge, a 75-year-old client in a skilled nursing facility, is 10 days status post pinning for a right femoral neck fracture. When you arrive at her room to bring her to therapy, Marge is lying in bed. Marge states that she just fell out of bed but was able to get back in bed by herself. She starts to cry and states, "I should not have told you I fell. I'm OK now. Please do not tell anyone what happened or they will put a restraint on me."

2. You are transferring a client from the hospital bed to a chair. The client is wearing only a hospital gown and is a little groggy from just waking up. As you are providing moderate assistance to transfer the client from sit to stand, the client suddenly becomes incontinent of feces, most of which lands directly on your shoe. The client does not appear to realize what just happened.

3. There are several clients present in the therapy room. As they are performing their exercises, they are making small talk and joking around. As the conversation turns to the topic of an upcoming election, the clients get into a very heated discussion and begin yelling at each other and using profanity.

4. A man receiving occupational therapy following a carpal tunnel release has been carrying a briefcase to each session. He typically asks for copies of his treatment notes and evaluations and places them in the briefcase. One day, when his treatment session has ended and the OTA is leaving the clinic to go to the occupational therapy office, the client calls the OTA back and says, "Look what I forgot to leave in my car." He then pulls out a handgun from the briefcase and turns it over several times to allow the OTA a good look.

5. A man is sent to occupational therapy directly from the physician's office for fabrication of a volar resting pan splint. The client had surgery 2 days ago to repair a lacerated extensor indicis tendon and had his surgical dressing removed moments ago. The OT realizes this appointment is urgent and squeezes the client into the therapist's busy, full work schedule today. However, the OT only has enough time to fabricate the splint and provide minimal instruction until the next day when the client will be scheduled for a full evaluation and follow-up splint check. The man is fitted with the splint and told not to remove it until he sees the OT tomorrow. However, the client does not show up the next day for his appointment. The OT calls to reschedule, but the client misses each appointment. Finally, after 2 weeks the client reappears complaining that his hand smells. The OT removes the splint and observes that the client's volar hand is severely macerated and the splint is soggy and odorous. When asked why this is, the client reported that he followed the OT's instruction not to remove his splint until he was seen back in therapy. In the meantime the client had bathed everyday with the splint on, not removing it to dry his skin.

Morreale, M. J. (2015). *Developing clinical competence: A workbook for the OTA*. Thorofare, NJ: SLACK Incorporated.

6. You are working in a skilled nursing facility with Harold, a 78-year-old client diagnosed with moderate stage Alzheimer's disease and a recent shoulder fracture. When you enter Harold's room to bring him to therapy, you discover that Harold has completely disrobed and is wandering around the room.

7. An OT working in an outpatient clinic fabricated a finger splint 2 days ago for a client. Today an OTA has been delegated this client for a follow-up splint check. When the client arrives, he reports that he accidentally flushed the splint down the toilet yesterday when washing his hands after toileting.

8. You are working in an outpatient clinic with a client who has a neurological condition. You transfer the client to the mat table in order to work on upper extremity exercises with the client positioned in supine. As the client initiates the exercises, you suddenly notice that the client was incontinent of urine, resulting in his pants and the mat getting wet. The client does not mention what just occurred.

9. You are a female OTA providing home care services to a young male client with a diagnosis of traumatic brain injury. Today you are alone in his basement apartment working with him on a dressing activity. Suddenly, the client reaches and grabs your breast.

10. You are working in an outpatient therapy clinic. One day you are sitting at a table with a client who is performing fine-motor activities. All of a sudden you notice that your client is slumped over and appears to be turning blue.

Debbie Amini, EdD, OTR/L, CHT, FAOTA has contributed significantly to this learning activity.

Learning Activity 8-7: Handling Situations Appropriately— More Practice

Indicate how you would respond appropriately with *professionalism and sensitivity* to the following actual clinical situations that various occupational therapy practitioners have encountered (identifying details have been changed). Consider what you would say to the clients, the immediate action you would take, and any follow-up that may be required.

1. Joe, a 55-year-old male client, has undergone hand surgery and is receiving outpatient occupational therapy. He has an outgoing personality, likes to make people laugh, and enjoys being the center of attention. Today there are five other middle-aged clients in the therapy clinic. Joe begins to loudly tell a joke that has sexual overtones.

2. A client is receiving outpatient occupational therapy following a shoulder fracture. The client has deep religious beliefs and always brings a Holy book to read in the clinic waiting room and during his hot pack treatments. Today the client inquires about the OTA's religious affiliation, which is very different than that of the client. The client states that the OTA is misguided and begins to proselytize. The client then asks the OTA to look at a passage in the Holy book.

3. An OTA is working with Stanley, a 75-year-old male who exhibits left hemiplegia and severe left neglect. As the OTA is walking past Stanley's hospital room, Stanley calls out excitedly for the OTA to come into his room right away. The OTA goes in his room and observes that Stanley is beaming. Stanley begins lifting his unaffected right arm and leg up and down vigorously while saying, "Look, look—it's a miracle! I can now move my arm and leg!"

4. An OTA working in a skilled nursing facility has been delegated a client who is diagnosed with chronic obstructive pulmonary disease. Today the client makes several derogatory remarks regarding the supervising OT's ethnicity (or religion) and then states, "Do I have to work with that OT? I would prefer to just work with you."

5. An OTA working in home care has been delegated a client, Eva, who is recovering from a hip fracture. Eva lives with her spouse and presently requires contact guard assistance to ambulate with a walker. As the OTA arrives at the client's home and is ringing the doorbell, the OTA can see Eva through the glass door panels. The OTA then observes that, as Eva starts to get up out of her chair unattended, she trips and falls to the floor. The client did not lose consciousness and calls out for help.

Morreale, M. J. (2015). *Developing clinical competence: A workbook for the OTA*. Thorofare, NJ: SLACK Incorporated.

Answers to Worksheets

Worksheet 8-1: Diseases

1. Trisomy 21—*Down syndrome*
2. Complex regional pain syndrome—*Reflex sympathetic dystrophy*
3. Lou Gehrig's disease—*Amyotrophic lateral sclerosis*
4. Herpes zoster—*Shingles*
5. Golfer's elbow—*Medial epicondylitis*
6. Degenerative joint disease—*Osteoarthritis*
7. Adhesive capsulitis—*Frozen shoulder*
8. Tennis elbow—*Lateral epicondylitis*
9. Gamekeeper's thumb—*Ulnar collateral ligament injury*
10. Epstein-Barr virus—*Mononucleosis*
11. Ewing sarcoma—*Bone cancer*
12. Barlow's syndrome—*Mitral valve prolapse*
13. Varicella—*Chickenpox*
14. Decubitus ulcer—*Pressure sore/bed sore*
15. Hypoglycemia—*Low blood sugar*
16. Myocardial infarction—*Heart attack*
17. Hypertension—*High blood pressure*
18. Hyperemesis—*Vomiting excessively*
19. Distal radius fracture—*Colle's fracture*
20. Hyperlipidemia—*Elevated lipid levels/high cholesterol*

Worksheet 8-2: Common Medications

Reference: Wilson, Shannon, & Shields, 2014

1. Warfarin—*Atrial fibrillation*
2. Nitroglycerin—*Angina*
3. Naproxen—*Osteoarthritis*
4. Aricept—*Dementia*
5. Risperdal—*Schizophrenia*
6. Atenolol—*Hypertension*
7. Diazepam—*Anxiety*
8. Boniva—*Osteoporosis*
9. Levodopa—*Parkinson's disease*
10. Topamax—*Seizure*
11. Demerol—*Pain*
12. Methotrexate—*Cancer*
13. Adderall—*Attention deficit disorder*
14. Lexapro—*Depression*
15. Proventil—*Asthma*
16. Augmentin—*Infection*
17. Avonex—*Multiple sclerosis*
18. Acyclovir—*Shingles*

19. Humulin R—*Diabetes*
20. Slow-FE—*Iron deficiency*

Worksheet 8-3: Generic Medications

Reference: Wilson et al., 2014

1. Warfarin—*Coumadin*
2. Omeprazole—*Prilosec*
3. Ibuprofen—*Advil*
4. Diazepam—*Valium*
5. Naproxen sodium—*Aleve*
6. Hydrocodone bitartrate—*Vicodin*
7. Albuterol—*Ventolin*
8. Gabapentin—*Neurontin*
9. Atorvastatin calcium—*Lipitor*
10. Clonazepam—*Klonopin*
11. Enalapril maleate—*Vasotec*
12. Alprazolam—*Xanax*
13. Insulin—*Humulin R*
14. Fluoxetine hydrochloride—*Prozac*
15. Diltiazem—*Cardizem*
16. Acetaminophen—*Tylenol*
17. Paroxetine—*Paxil*
18. Duloxetine hydrochloride—*Cymbalta*
19. Calcium carbonate—*Tums*
20. Atenolol—*Tenormin*

Worksheet 8-4: *Occupational Therapy Practice Framework*

Some items fit neatly into one category, whereas other activities may be placed into several different categories depending on the particular context and one's personal values, interests, or roles (AOTA, 2014). For example, reading email can be a work-related task, a leisurely way to pass time, or considered a means of social communication. Thus, your classifications may be slightly different than the ones indicated below.

Client Activity	BADL	IADL	Play	Leisure	Work	Education	Rest and Sleep	Social Participation
Baking bread		*		*				
Cleaning contact lenses	*							
Taking the train to get to a job		*						
Donning a splint	*							
Playing hopscotch with others			*					
Attending religious services								*
Making a collage for an OTA class homework assignment						*		

Client Activity	BADL	IADL	Play	Leisure	Work	Education	Rest and Sleep	Social Participation
Watching TV to fall asleep				*			*	
Feeding the household cat or dog		*						
Listening to music				*				
Preparing a résumé					*			
Functional ambulation	*							
Taking a nap							*	
Babysitting a younger sibling		*			*			*
Organizing school papers into folders						*		
Volunteering at a hospital gift shop					*			*
Attending a bridal shower or bachelor party								*
Paying bills		*						
Getting to next class on time						*		
Knitting a sweater to wear				*				
Using contraception	*							*
Setting an alarm clock							*	
Reading emails				*	*			*
Taking vitamins		*						
Sewing a button back on a shirt		*						
Planting flowers in the yard		*		*				
Writing a performance review for a staff member					*			
Navigating a wheelchair in the home	*							
Dressing a doll			*					
Exercising at the gym		*		*				
Calling 911 when smelling smoke		*						
Eating lunch with colleagues				*	*			*

Worksheet 8-5: Grading and Adapting—Making Coffee

Here are some suggestions although you may come up with others. Consider which modifications are needed due to motor difficulties versus cognitive impairment.

Activity Demand: Task Material—Coffee	Activity Demand: Required Action of Opening Coffee Container	Activity Demand: Required Action of Measuring Coffee	Activity Demand: Required Action of Heating the Water/Brewing Coffee
Example: Instant coffee	*Example: Can of coffee requiring use of a can opener*	*Example: Use a measuring spoon*	*Example: Boil water in teakettle using stove*
Whole coffee beans Coffee "teabags" Specific type of coffee (decaffeinated vs. regular, espresso-type coffee, flavored) Bottle of liquid iced coffee Ground coffee	Jar with lid Tear off pouch Cut pouch with scissors Box/carton (pods) Screw cap/bottle top Can of coffee with a metal/foil pull-off lid Can of coffee with a plastic lid Place coffee in another container or bag Carafe/thermos (containing hot coffee)	Single-serve instant coffee packet Pods/K-cups Premeasured drip coffee package Have family member pre-measure and place in plastic bags or containers	Microwave water Electric kettle/hot pot with/without automatic shut-off Automatic drip coffee maker with/without automatic shut-off Programmable machine family member can preset Espresso/cappuccino machine K-cup machine Electric percolator Stovetop glass percolator Stovetop metal percolator (espresso) French press

Worksheet 8-6: Grading and Adapting—Laundry

List the sequence of steps to wash clothes and ways to grade and adapt each step. You may come up with other suggestions.

Sequence of Steps to Perform the Occupation of Laundry	Grade/Adapt Task Methods	Grade/Adapt Task Materials
Example: Carry a laundry basket full of clothes	*Example: Place dirty clothes directly in machine when getting changed*	*Example: Use a rolling laundry cart* *Use a laundry bag*
Check pockets before putting clothes in laundry basket	Post visual reminders	Wear clothing without pockets
Sort items (by color, materials delicate, hand-wash)	Post list of instructions Sit instead of stand	Use a divided laundry cart

Sequence of Steps to Perform the Occupation of Laundry	Grade/Adapt Task Methods	Grade/Adapt Task Materials
Open machine lid/door and put appropriate amount of items in machine	Take clothes to dry cleaner Use a laundry service Use a hamper or basket to determine correct amount of laundry to put in machine Sit instead of stand	Use a reacher Use a front-loading versus a top-loading machine Use a coin-operated machine
Open detergent containers and measure detergent, fabric softener, bleach (pour into cap, use scoop measure)	Use premeasured detergent or pods Use markings on caps	Premeasured detergent/pods Use dispenser type bottle Laundry detergent sheets Powder versus liquid Dryer sheets Use a different measuring device Purchase items from laundromat vending machine Use small-sized containers
Put detergent, bleach, softener in proper machine dispensers and close lid	Label dispensers clearly	Pod or detergent sheet versus liquid or powder Use an "all in one" product Use small-sized containers
Set proper cycles temp, delicate/heavy-duty, fabric softener, extra rinse and turn machine on	Post list of instructions Label cycles clearly	Use machine with more or less buttons or cycles Push buttons, digital panel, or a dial
Remember to take clothes out of machine	Designate a consistent day and time to do laundry Stay by machine to perform other tasks	Machine with an audible signal Use a timer
Put clothes in dryer and set time/setting on dryer	Sit instead of stand Hang up clothes instead Post list of instructions	Clothesline Drying rack Use a reacher Use a machine with less buttons or cycles
Remember to take clothes out of machine and put away	Store clothing close to washer and dryer	Machine with an audible signal Use a timer Use a reacher

Worksheet 8-7: Billing and Reimbursement

Suggested resources: Morreale & Borcherding, 2013; Thomas, 2011

The AOTA website (www.AOTA.org) has useful information about public policy and reimbursement of occupational therapy services. Further information about Medicare can be found at www.medicare.gov, and information about Medicaid can be found at www.medicaid.gov. The CMS manuals can be found online at www.cms.gov. Publication 100-02: Medicare Benefit Policy Manual (Chapter 15, Section 220) delineates the criteria for reimbursement of outpatient occupational therapy services.

1. A. According to the CMS guidelines for co-treating, the total units billed by both disciplines cannot exceed the allowable units based on time: 30 minutes equals 2 units. The OTA and PTA can each bill 1 unit or *either* the OTA or PTA can bill the entire 2 units (CMS, 2009).

2. A. According to CMS, 1 unit of a timed service equals 8 to 22 minutes (CMS, 2011).

3. B. Medicare Part A covers inpatient acute stays, although there are some out-of-pocket expenses.

4. A. Inpatient hospital stays using Medicare Part A is reimbursed through the Prospective Payment System, which pays a predetermined per-diem rate.

5. B. The client has to pay the full cost of the deductible before the insurance provides any reimbursement. To meet the deductible, the client has to pay in full for the evaluation ($100), plus $50 for the second visit. For the remaining $20 owed for the second visit, the insurance pays 80% ($16) and the patient must pay the remaining $4. Thus, the total out-of-pocket cost for the second visit is $54 ($50 + $4).

6. D. TRICARE is health insurance for military members and their family. Unemployment insurance covers some lost wages, but does not reimburse health care costs. Medicare is a separate program.

7. C. Answers A, B, and D are classified as durable medical equipment. Items such as tub seats, grab bars, reachers, sock aids, and the like are not, as they are considered self-help or hygienic devices and not considered medical in nature (CMS, 2005).

8. C. IDEA Part C covers children under 3 years of age. IDEA Part B covers preschool and school-aged children (National Dissemination Center for Children with Disabilities, 2011).

9. D. Medicaid covers health care costs for eligible individuals who meet low-income guidelines. Unemployment insurance, Supplemental Security Insurance, and Workers' Compensation are separate programs that do not cover health care costs.

10. C. CPT is billing codes for health care services provided. ICD-10 contains diagnosis codes. The Minimum Data Set is an assessment tool used in skilled nursing facilities. The client is not likely eligible for Medicare.

Worksheet 8-8: Department Management

Suggested resources: Ellexson, 2011; Giles, 2011

- *Space:* Here are suggestions when choosing a space but you may come up with others:
  - o Meets requirements for local zoning and building codes
  - o Available client base in area
  - o Proximity to competitors in area
  - o Wheelchair accessibility
  - o Parking
  - o Space adequate for types of services to be provided/number of rooms
  - o Outdoor facilities/space if required (e.g., playground equipment for sensory integration or gross-motor tasks)
  - o Bathroom facilities present in space or building
  - o Adequate electrical outlets and supply
  - o Adequate water supply for hand hygiene, splinting, etc.
  - o Overhead lighting
- *Equipment and supplies:* The specific equipment and supplies required will depend on the type of practice setting, space, and available budget. Some considerations are noted below.
  - o Safety—Personal protective equipment (e.g., gloves, gown, mask), fire extinguisher, smoke detector, soap and paper towels, first aid kit, wheelchair, etc.

o Office furniture—Chairs, desk, table, mat, plinth, etc.

o Office equipment—Computer, phone, fax, copier, file cabinets, washer/dryer, etc.

o Office supplies—Pens, paper, toner, envelopes, stapler, paper clips, folders, etc.

o Evaluation tools—Specific formal/informal assessments, goniometer, tape measure, dynamometer, pinch meter, volumeter, specific sensory tests, etc.

o General supplies—Bandages, treatment table paper, pillows, pillowcases, towels, crayons, toys, lotion, etc.

o Exercise equipment—Putty, weights, exercise bands, pegboard, cones, hand grippers, etc.

o Physical agent modalities—Paraffin unit, paraffin, hydrocollator, hot packs, cold packs, terrycloth covers, tongs, timer, etc.

o ADL equipment—Refrigerator, stove, microwave, coffee maker, laundry basket, pots/pans, utensils, etc.

o Adaptive equipment—Reachers, buttonhooks, long-handle shoehorns, built-up utensils, etc.

o Splinting supplies—Splint pan, heat gun, thermoplastics, hook and loop fastener, scissors, spatula, pre-fabricated splints, etc.

- *Possible staff or professional services needed (non-inclusive list):*
  o Accountant
  o Attorney
  o Janitor/handyman
  o Cleaning person
  o Electrician/plumber/carpenter (will depend on renovations required)
  o Engineering service/technician to calibrate or repair medical equipment
  o Billing service
  o Secretary
  o Marketing professional/web designer
  o Information technology specialist
  o Landscaper/snow removal
  o Rehabilitation aide
  o Laundry service

Worksheet 8-9: Budget

Reference: Ellexson, 2011

1. F. A fiscal year goes from January 1 to December 31.
   An organization determines its own fiscal time frame consisting of a 1-year period, such as October 1 to September 30.

2. F. An example of an occupational therapy capital budget expenditure is a tub seat.
   A capital expense is a larger cost item, such as items >$1000, that can be considered an asset and usually depreciated. A tub seat comes under the category of general equipment and supplies and does not meet those criteria.

3. F. Revenue equals total income minus expenses.
   Revenue equals total income before expenses.

4. T. An example of a fixed cost is rent.
   Fixed costs are steady for a period of time and not impacted by volume of services.

5. T. Accounts receivable include the money due from an insurance company.

6. T. An example of variable expenses are office supplies.

7. F. Nonprofit means that the organization does not meet its expenses.

8. T. Total costs subtracted from revenue equals profits.

9. F. An occupational therapy department budget always contains money for staff to attend continuing education seminars to maintain NBCOT certification.

10. T. Costs for items ordered but not paid for are considered accounts payable.

11. T. Bandages, lotions, and paraffin are considered direct use supplies.

12. F. Cash flow consists of pending money due from third-party payers.
    Cash flow is the money that actually comes in and out and is available for use.

13. T. Expenses that are fixed, such as salaries and equipment leases, are called overhead.

14. T. Productivity refers to the amount of billable services that an individual provides.

15. T. A piece of capital equipment that is depreciating is considered an asset.

References

American Academy of Professional Coders. (2014). *In the news.* Retrieved from www.aapc.com/index.php/2014/05/in-the-news/

American Occupational Therapy Association. (2010a). Occupational therapy code of ethics and ethics standards (2010). *American Journal of Occupational Therapy, 64*(6 Suppl.), S17-S26. doi: 10.5014/ajot.2010.64S17

American Occupational Therapy Association. (2010b). Standards of practice for occupational therapy. *American Journal of Occupational Therapy, 64*(6 Suppl.), S106-S111. doi: 10.5014/ajot.2010.64S106

American Occupational Therapy Association. (2014). Occupational therapy practice framework: Domain and process (3rd ed.). *American Journal of Occupational Therapy, 68*(1 Suppl.), S1-S48. doi: 10.5014/ajot.2014.682006

Centers for Medicare & Medicaid Services. (2005). *Medicare national coverage determinations (NCD) manual* (Pub. 100-03: Ch 1, section 280.1). Baltimore, MD: Centers for Medicare & Medicaid Services. Retrieved from www.cms.gov/Regulations-and-Guidance/Guidance/Manuals/Internet-Only-Manuals-IOMs-Items/CMS014961.html

Centers for Medicare & Medicaid Services. (2009). *11 Part B billing scenarios for PTs and OTs.* Retrieved from www.cms.gov/Medicare/Billing/TherapyServices/downloads/11_Part_B_Billing_Scenarios_for_PTs_and_OTs.pdf

Centers for Medicare & Medicaid Services. (2011). *Medicare claims processing manual* (Pub. 100-04: Ch 5, section 20.2). Baltimore, MD: Centers for Medicare & Medicaid Services. Retrieved from www.cms.gov/Regulations-and-Guidance/Guidance/Manuals/downloads//clm104c05.pdf

Ellexson, M. T. (2011). Financial planning and budgeting. In K. Jacobs & G. L. McCormack (Eds.), *The occupational therapy manager* (5th ed.) (pp. 113-125). Bethesda, MD: American Occupational Therapy Association.

Giles, G. M. (2011). Starting a new program, business, or practice. In K. Jacobs & G. L. McCormack (Eds.), *The occupational therapy manager* (5th ed.) (pp. 145-166). Bethesda, MD: American Occupational Therapy Association.

Morreale, M. J., & Borcherding, S. (2013). *The OTA's guide to documentation: Writing SOAP notes* (3rd ed.). Thorofare, NJ: SLACK Incorporated.

National Dissemination Center for Children with Disabilities. (2011). *Part C of IDEA: Early intervention for babies and toddlers.* Retrieved from http://nichcy.org/laws/idea/partc

Thomas, J. V. (2011). Reimbursement. In K. Jacobs & G. L. McCormack (Eds.), *The occupational therapy manager* (5th ed.) (pp. 385-405). Bethesda, MD: American Occupational Therapy Association.

Wilson, B. A., Shannon, M. T., & Shields, K. M. (2014). *Pearson nurse's drug guide.* Upper Saddle River, NJ: Pearson Education, Inc.

World Health Organization. (2013). *Classifications: International classification of diseases (ICD) information sheet.* Geneva: Author. Retrieved from www.who.int/classifications/icd/factsheet/en/index.html

Index